Breast Health and Bra Comfort

Geoff Kirby

Copyright © 2014 Geoff Kirby

All rights reserved.

ISBN-10: 1497582792
ISBN-13: 978-1497582798

CONTENTS

Acknowledgments   i

1 **Introduction.** Why 80% of women wear badly fitting bras and what the consequences may be. Going bra-less is an option that should be tried for a few months   1

2 **Does Bra Wearing Create Health Problems?** There is no evidence that bra wearing offers any health benefits but there is much evidence that bras in general, and badly fitting bras in particular, cause significant, possibly life threatening health problems.   9

3 **Comparison Of Online Bra Fitting Guides.** Conclusion? They are overwhelmingly useless and most are putting women's health at risk.   41

4 **The 'Portsmouth' Study.** A large study involving forty-five women who had their bras checked against a traditional sizing method and found most were wearing very much the wrong bra sizes.   51

5 **A New Bra Sizing Scheme.** Time to sweep away existing bra sizing schemes that don't work. A new and better bra sizing system is described.   57

6 **How Does A Bra Work?** How do bras work and what do you need to know when buying one?   63

7 **Bra Buying Problems.** Bras with the same size on the label can vary enormously in actual band and cup size making it very difficult to buy bras that fit. Wrong bra sizes are deliberately sewn into the bras.   67

8 **Pulling It All Together.** What you have learned. Spread the word!   75

9 **About The Author.** Why a sixty year interest in breasts qualifies me to write this book.   79

10 **Further Reading**   81

11 **References.**   83

The Propaganda

'Not wearing a bra causes sagging. Girls should be measured from age nine onwards throughout their lives for bras. There is no other way to keep breast shape in later life'

Playtex expert trainer teaching bra fitting consultants (2000)

The Admission.

'We have no medical evidence that a bra can prevent sagging'

John Dixey General Manager Playtex (2000)

The Scientific Evidence

Wearing a bra makes sagging worse. Going bra-less reduces sagging, firms the breasts, reduces breast pain and the effects of cysts and may also reduce vulnerability to breast cancer. Any advantage from wearing a bra is psychological and created by a massive bra industry advertising campaign.

The Recommendation

Give up your bra for a few weeks and feel the benefits. If you don't like it simply put on your bra again - or better still buy a new bra selected using the advice in this book. You have nothing to lose and possibly a lot to gain!

ACKNOWLEDGMENTS

Copyright of the text and photographs resides with the author except where pictures have been attributed to Wiki Commons Media or to Mr David Moth.

I have unlimited praise for the support of my partner throughout this labour. She has never said *'You love that laptop more than you love me!'* and has been a willing photographic model, proof reader and friend.

I also gratefully express the support and help given by Dr Jenny White of Portsmouth University. Not only did she generously make available the data she and Dr Joanna Scurr collected but she gave valuable guidance.

Mr David Moth was very helpful by bringing my attention to the work of Sydney Ross Singer and Soma Grismaijer published in their books *'Dressed To Kill'* and *'Get It Off!'* as well as 2000 Channel 4 documentary *'Bras: The Bare Truth'*. David also allowed me to use his photograph as well as his measurements of bra pressure on the breast.

My author website is www.geoffkirby.co.uk/Books

'I have suffered from fibrocystic breasts my entire adult life. At age 52, the lumps in my breasts had become so numerous, large and painful I could no longer ignore them.

'After doing some research online, I stopped wearing a bra. After about a week the pain and tenderness disappeared and now, four months later, the lumps have all gone away with none taking their place. This result has been dramatic and transformational for me.

'I wanted to share it with other women since this is a very common condition.

'Needless to say, this treatment costs nothing and has no side effects. I wish my doctor had told me about this.'

Anonymous blogger

'The People's Pharmacy' http://tinyurl.com/3vl8q86

1. INTRODUCTION

This book will explain why 80% of women wear bras that don't fit properly and why the majority of these wearers will suffer breast pain; sometimes so severely as to seriously affect their lifestyles.

It has been suggested that wearing badly fitting bras may cause breast cancer although this is still a highly contentious issue eighteen years after the survey was published that gave rise to this claim. [1]

Chapter 2 starts this examination of the bra wearing habit by critically summarising the health issues claimed for strapping your breasts into a bra.

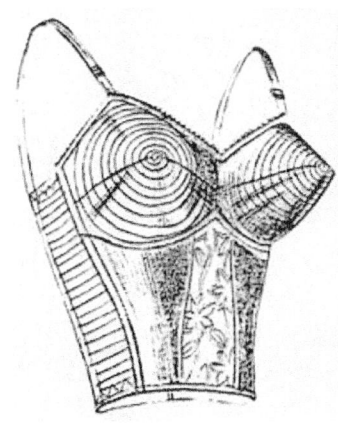

OMG! Was this 1950s bra ever going to be comfortable? [2]

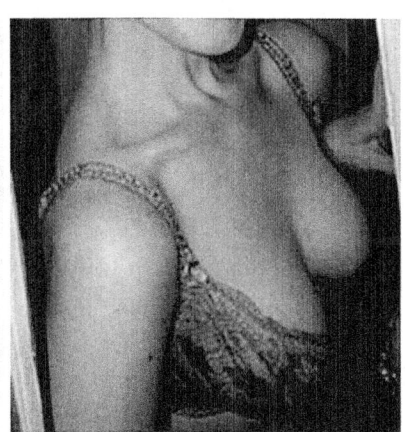

That's better! [3]

INTRODUCTION

Perhaps surprisingly, it has been found that wearing a bra actually increases sagging. Indeed, measurements on women who go bra-less show that sagging is less than for women who habitually wear bras.

In a medical study in which one hundred women wore their normal bras for three months then went bra-less for three months, the pre-menstrual women suffering moderate or severe breast pain found that the number of days of pain was halved when bra-less. Overall, for all the women, there was an increase of 7% in days when pain was absent.

As volunteers in the study stated

'I've been given back my freedom. Breast pain has gone, my worry has stopped and I'm enjoying life more.'

'The trial was magic! I'll never go back to wearing a bra.'

'I used to think of my bras as 'Comfort, Control and Support' but now I see them as 'Contain, Restrain and Complain'.

Apart from cystic pain problems bras can just be a pain because the underwires and straps cut into delicate flesh and leave deep red wheals on the ribcage or shoulders.

If you are still having periods the recommendation emerging from chapter 2 is to try going bra-less for a month or two. If you have breast pain or pain specifically associated with cysts then you have a good chance of gaining significant relief and your breasts will not head south.

The claim that bra wearing can cause breast cancer is contentious and much disputed. The claims and counter-claims are discussed in chapter 2.

Despite the considerable health advantages of going bra-less it is a habit that the overwhelming majority of women will not give up. This is because the vastly powerful bra industry advertises their bras on their sex appeal and not on their comfort or health properties.

Pressure groups that try to persuade women to go bra-less are pushing on a locked door. People smoke, drink alcohol, wear stiletto heeled shoes - all knowing the health risks. They are balancing the pleasure against the pain and opting for the pleasure; in the case of bras it is the dubious notion of looking 'sexier'.

INTRODUCTION

Why do 80% of bra-wearing women end up wearing a badly fitting, painful and - possibly - health threatening bra?

One reason is their reluctance to part with an old friend. I'm sure that some women simply do not think about throwing out a bra that is long past its prime with saggy cups, overstretched straps and broken hooks. The appearance created by an ill-fitting bra can be unflattering at best and positively disgusting at worst - think the 'Fat Slags' from VIZ [4] if you need persuading to buy a new bra!

Another reason for badly fitting bras being so widespread is that online bra fitting guides give spectacularly inaccurate advice on bra size.

My partner's most consistently comfortable bra size is 36B. Using a large number of online bra fitting advice websites I found that the range of advised sizes for her measurements was as widely varied as 38AA, 38D and 34DD! None of the twenty-one online guides checked predicted a size 36B as the best fit.

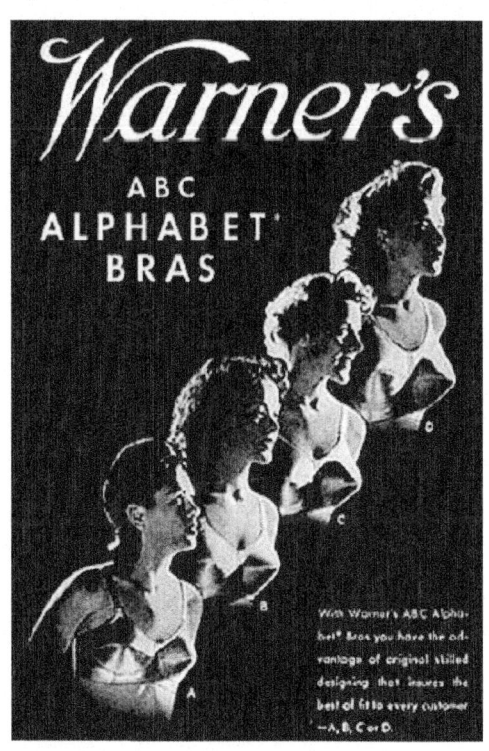

An advertisement by Warner (1944) [5].

INTRODUCTION

We will see in chapter 3 that online bra fitting guides are so unreliable that women who buy online frequently discover that the bra that arrives in the post is nowhere near as comfortable as the bra which had been an old friend for years.

Having tried on the newly delivered ill-fitting bra there is a dilemma. Go to all the trouble of returning it and probably getting back an equally poorly fitting bra, wearing it and putting up with the bad painful fit or abandoning it to the back of the underwear drawer along with all the other bras and knickers which should have been thrown away years ago.

On the Ann Summers website we can read [6]

'It's time to say goodbye to bad bras! All you need to do is combine both your measurements (Bust and Under Bust) to find the right bra size on the chart.'

If only that were true!

The Figleaves website [7] and Bravissimo website [8] give sensible guides to bra buying. They ask the user to wear her most comfortable bra and then answer a detailed multi-choice questionnaire about any faults in the fit. From these answers and the size of the bra being worn an alternative size is recommended.

To be fair, online bra retailers mostly (but not always) say that bras need to be tried on in the presence of a professional bra fitter to get a satisfactory fit. But isn't that defeating the convenience of online shopping for a bra?

How many fulltime mums and professional women have the time to make appointments to have such a fitting especially when stores in small towns may not be offering this service?

This is why a survey in 2012 [9] found that over two-thirds of women had never used a bra fitting service.

Even when professional bra fitters are used they sometimes persuade a customer to buy an ill-fitting bra because the size required is not available in store at that time.

One online bra selling website even suggests that sharing a cubicle with a stranger may be unsafe and that is why their online bra service should be used! Has anyone ever encountered a perverted bra fitter?

Chapter 4 discusses a fascinating study conducted at Portsmouth

INTRODUCTION

University in the UK where forty five volunteers were asked the size of their most comfortable bra. These ladies were then professionally measured and fitted with a good bra. It was found that these women predominantly over-estimated their correct bra band size by as much as six inches and consistently underestimated their correct cup size such that one lady who thought she was a 'B' cup size was measured and found to be a 'G'!

Chapter 5 offers a brand new bra sizing scheme invented by me which is much more accurate than the existing mishmash of hopelessly inaccurate online guides.

My new scheme should get you within a band and cup size of your comfortable size. This is much better than the many existing online bra fitting guides which can be as much as four inches out on band size and four cup sizes in error.

This will be a boon to both online sellers and buyers resulting in many fewer returns from frustrated customers.

Chapter 6 explains how a bra works by deconstructing it into its parts and showing what to check out in a good bra.

Chapter 7 shows that bras are made to different shapes and sizes even though they carry the same sizes on the labels. Modern bras are labelled with smaller back sizes and larger cup sizes than a decade or so ago so that the wearer is flattered into thinking that she is not only slimmer, but larger in the bust.

This is known as *'Vanity Sizing'* and it is rampant in the sizing of dresses as well as bras. A lady tries on a dress size smaller than her usual size - and it fits! The manufacturer of that dress believes the woman will be delighted that she has gone down a dress size and will come back again for her next dress.

Are women really that silly?

Of course not!

However, in the male dominated, misogynistic world of clothing manufacturing and marketing, the bra buying woman is still treated as a fool. The result is that bras carrying the same size on the label can vary by up to two band sizes and two cup sizes from each other. One bra will be baggy and hopeless whilst another will be impossible to clasp at the back even though they have the same size printed on the label.

Branding the system 'a scam', New York boutique owner Linda

INTRODUCTION

Becker says women who have not been fitted for some time could easily be wearing a poorly-fitting bra because many manufacturers have changed the sizing without warning customers.

In an interview with ABC News, Ms Becker, who calls herself 'The Bra Lady', said:

'I realized all the companies about 10 years ago changed all the sizes without telling us. They 'vanity sized' it. They wanted you to think your back was smaller and your breasts were bigger.'

Describing the scale of the problem, she says that what was once labelled a 36D in the USA is now often labelled a 32G.

A survey carried out by the UK newspaper Mail Online [10] sent a lady wearing a comfortable 32C bra to a number of shops to be professionally fitted with a new bra and found out that few 32C bras were suitable and the most comfortable bras ranged from 30D to 34C depending on the bra manufacturer. This proves that even bras of nominally the same size vary enormously in both band size and cup size.

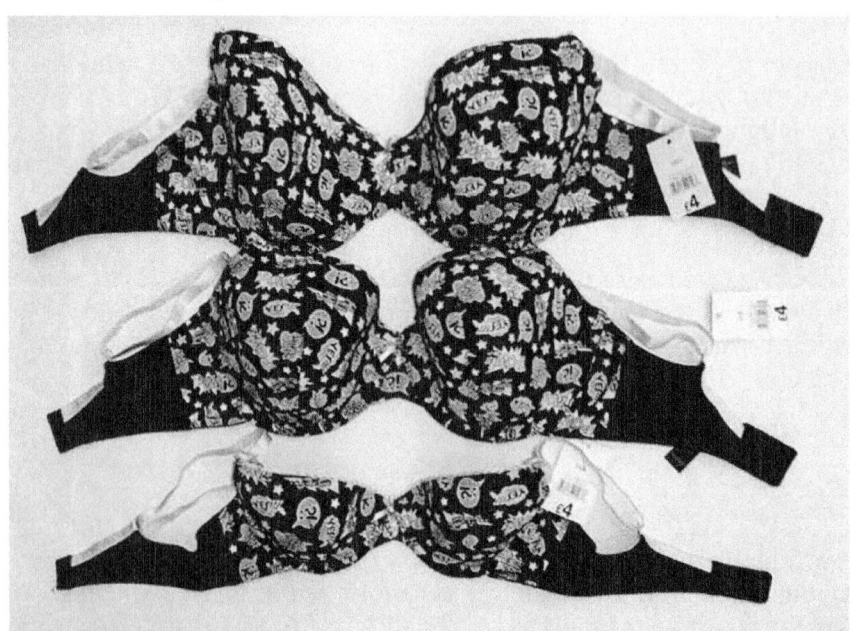

The above picture shows three bras of the same make and style. Their sizes are 34A, 34E and 34G from bottom to top.

Because the band sizes are the same, all bra buying guides say that they will fit women with the same under-bust (rib cage)

INTRODUCTION

measurement. It is obvious from the picture that this is not true. The 34A bra measured 25.2 inches from hooks to eyes unstretched whilst the 34G bra measured 28.0 inches.

The following [11] are typical quotes from women who have suffered the consequences of wholly inaccurate bra sizing guides, mediocre advice from bra fitting professionals and bras carrying incorrect sizes on their labels.

'My whole life I've had one good bra - one bra that was comfortable, that didn't leave enormous scarlet wheals on my flesh that gave me two breasts instead of one; that gave support without stopping me breathing. One good bra!'

'It was a sort of blue pebbledash cotton thing from Sock Shop and I kept it going for five years. It was disgustingly unattractive, but under clothes my breasts looked like my breasts when I was wearing it. I cried when the much darned strap finally gave in last year and I had to throw it out. Since then I've bought about one bra a week and none of them are comfortable. All of them leave marks.'

'I went out dancing once, sporting an all-new underwired number and returned home to find huge parts of my chest gouged out by evil, satanic wiring. I think this might be one of the consequences of wearing such items if one is not overly endowed.'

'I nagged my mother for a little black satin number for my 18th birthday. I tried to ignore the unarguable truth that it gave me a comedy trapezium-shaped bust and no cleavage to speak of. I felt like an utter fraud all night and suffered nasty red strap-marks on my shoulders where I had winched up the bra in an attempt to gain cleavage. It's really not surprising that I should favour vests now, is it?"

If your bras cut in and you can't find a bra that fits you are in the majority. Read the story on one woman's *'Battle With The Bras'* and know that you are not alone! [12]

Ladies! You deserve better from your bras!

Chapter 8 'pulls it all together' by summarising what you have learned. You will now understand the claims and counter-claims about the health risks of wearing a bra, realise that the reason comfortable bras are so difficult to buy is because the bra sizing guides are useless and the bras themselves are often 'vanity sized' meaning that the wrong sizes are printed on the labels to convince

INTRODUCTION

you that you are slimmer than you thought and that your breasts are bigger and hence 'sexier'.

The bra manufacturers and retailers are putting the health of your breasts at risk with their Machiavellian tactics which are for one purpose only - to make vast profits.

Don't let them get away with it!

DID YOU KNOW THAT…

…in the 1960s there was a popular party game in which ladies attempted to hold a pencil under their bare breasts without it dropping. Known as 'The Pencil Test' it was proudly used by young ladies to demonstrate to their audience of appreciative young men that their breasts were not 'saggy'.

DID YOU KNOW THAT…

…the word 'brassiere' means 'under arm'? It was first included in the 1912 Oxford English Dictionary.

2. DOES BRA WEARING CREATE HEALTH PROBLEMS?

"It is a capital mistake to theorize before you have all the evidence. It biases the judgement."

— Sir Arthur Conan Doyle, *'A Study in Scarlet'*

Is there a breast illness epidemic?

Women in Britain buy each year about 75 million bras worth £500 million. In the USA sales run at about $5 billion each year.

Seven per cent of women in the UK suffer from cysts and most of them wear bras.

Breast cancer incidence rates per head of population in Britain are two-thirds higher today than they were thirty years ago and seven times greater than a century ago.

Clinical breast pain is suffered by 40% of women in the UK although many simply put up with this condition and never report it believing it to be an inconvenience that women are required to suffer to avoid the indignity of breasts drooping if the bra is rejected [13].

Could there be a connection between breast pain, cysts, breast cancer and wearing a bra? Many people claim there is such a connection whilst the majority of medical experts say that these claims are unfounded and alarmist.

This chapter attempts to set out the evidence in an accessible form.

DOES BRA WEARING CREATE HEALTH PROBLEMS?

Discussing health issues associated with wearing bras is dangerous terrain for a male pensioner in his seventy-fifth year with no medical training.

However I worked for 45 years as a professional scientist, I have two university degrees in science topics and my career speciality has been in analysing data to make judgements in complex situations. I hope my views here can make a valid contribution to the important issue of women's breast health.

The first important conclusion is that I have found no evidence that wearing bras is beneficial apart from a proportion of women who believe that bra wearing is 'uplifting' to the soul as well as the breasts. The soul may well be uplifted but the breasts still sag with age.

Is 'Lifting and Squeezing' the breasts good for them?

This is a deep question heavily coloured by cultural influences going back into to prehistory.

The reason why human females have larger breasts than other primates is still a mystery. Desmond Morris pointed out that female gorillas are pretty much flat chested [14] and yet can suckle infants just as well as human females with large bulbous breasts.

Human females did not evolve large breasts to suckle hungry babies. There was an unrelated reason for those mammary swellings unique in the primate world.

Morris suspected that large human female breasts evolved when our ancestors changed from rear entry sex to front entry; the breasts then evolved to appear similar to the buttocks as a sexual enticement symbol.

Things have moved on since then with competing theories about the origins of breasts as sex symbols.

However, it is still a popular dogma with evolutionary scientists that human breasts are potent sex symbols that are powerful incentives to attract a mate. Thumbing through men's so-called 'adult' magazines seems to confirm this idea although I fail to understand why any woman would consider the size of her cleavage to be reliable means of finding that 'sincere, caring soul mate with GSOH' so widely sought on dating websites and in magazines.

For an excellent and amusing account of the role of human breasts

DOES BRA WEARING CREATE HEALTH PROBLEMS?

in historical and modern times read Florence Williams' *'Breasts: Natural and Unnatural History'* which is available from Amazon [15].

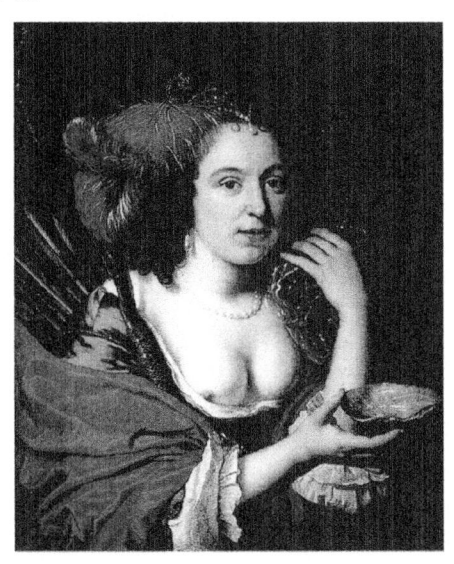

A desirable full busted woman from the 1660s [16]

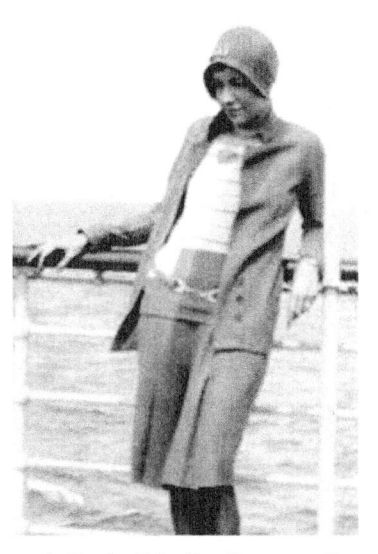

A desirable flat breasted woman from the 1920s [17]

Why then were men so attracted to full busted women before the 1920s but then attracted to flat chested women in the 1920s? What happened around 1920?

Don't the changes in men's interest in women's breasts over the centuries indicate that breasts have not been universally potent sexual symbols?

If it were true that breasts have, in the long-term, been sexual symbols then why have breasts not evolved to be the perfection of every man's sexual fantasies?

A few years ago an evolutionary biologist went on UK television to predict that, within one thousand years, humans will have rapidly evolved by natural sexual selection to the 'ideal' shapes meaning slim blonde women with size DD breasts and men with large penises.

What nonsense!

If evolution were to create these Stepford Men and Women it would have happened long ago.

DOES BRA WEARING CREATE HEALTH PROBLEMS?

But look around!

Flat chested women clearly have no problem finding loving men with large penises.

Bra cup sizes range from size AA to size N.

For that matter penises also show enormous variations amongst men [18].

Breast and penis sizes are clearly not a significant factor in choosing a mate. If they were, breasts and penises would long ago have evolved rapidly to the optimum attractive size - just as peacock's tails have evolved to the optimum size compromising between sexual attractiveness and the ability to move around, eat and mate.

Ladies, if you cannot give up your bras then buy bras that are comfortable and healthy without dreaming that your ideal lover's thoughts will be dominated with the shape and size of your breasts.

You should be loved for who you are not for the size and shape of your breasts or the name on the label of your designer bra. After, all, if you believe that a lover is attracted by your bra what will happen when it is removed to reveal...

No - let's change the subject!

Do bras stop sagging breasts?

Sagging with age is a natural function accelerated by smoking, number of pregnancies, tendency to obesity and age. There is also no evidence that breastfeeding causes breasts to head south [19].

Perhaps surprisingly, it has been found that wearing a bra actually increases sagging.

Measurements on women who go bra-less show that sagging is less than for women who habitually wear bras. In a 15-year study [20] by the University of Besançon in eastern France, sports science Professor Jean-Denis Rouillon found that wearing a bra may not keep a woman's breasts from sagging nor alleviate back pain.

The researchers found that the nipples of women who didn't wear bras didn't head south but actually *lifted* an average of 7 millimetres toward the shoulders in a year and the breasts became firmer.

DOES BRA WEARING CREATE HEALTH PROBLEMS?

Jean-Denis Rouillon reported

'Medically, physiologically, anatomically - breasts gain no benefit from being denied gravity. On the contrary, they get saggier with a bra.'

Stretching of the breast ligaments and drooping in later life is a function of the weight of heavy breasts and not whether a bra is worn.

Increased risk of breast cancer - 'Dressed to Kill'

The book 'Dressed to Kill' proposed a claim pursued by Sydney Ross Singer and Soma Grismaijer since the mid-1990s [21] that bra wearing increases substantially the chance of suffering breast cancer and that the mechanism is through bra pressure impeding the working of the lymphatic system in the breasts.

The work of Singer and Grismaijer follows two threads.

The first thread is a survey of women's bra wearing habits with and without breast cancer. The number of hours spent each day wearing a bra before the cancer was diagnosed was found to correlate with the proportion of women with breast cancer. The authors went on to conclude that bra wearing causes breast cancer.

The second thread is that the pressure exerted by bras interferes with the lymphatic system in and around the ribcage and this reduces the ability of the lymphatic system to drain away toxins and encourages breast cancer to form.

On their blog they blame '*...backed-up fluid which results in cysts and pain.*

'This stagnant lymph fluid cannot be adequately flushed away, concentrating waste products and toxins in the slowly toxifying breasts. Ultimately, this can lead to cancer.'

This interpretation of the results of their survey has met with almost universal denial by the medical profession.

The authors of 'Dressed To Kill' write

'To the industry that makes billions of dollars each year giving mammograms, mastectomies, radiation and chemotherapies, and then prostheses and bras so these women can look 'normal', the concept of bras contributing to breast cancer is absurd'.

DOES BRA WEARING CREATE HEALTH PROBLEMS?

It is no surprise that a very large number of women have become alarmed that bra wearing may increase their risk of suffering breast cancer especially when there is no evidence that being bra-free is a problem.

However, typical of the opponents of this hypothesis is the following opinion published in the New York Times in 2010. Dr. Ted Gansler, director of medical content for the American Cancer Society wrote

'There is no scientifically credible evidence (that bra wearing can cause cancer), he said, and the proposed mechanism — that bras prevent elimination of toxins by blocking lymph flow — is not in line with scientific concepts of how breast cancer develops.

Because the idea of bras causing breast cancer is so scientifically implausible, it seems unlikely that researchers will ever spend their time and resources to test it in a real epidemiological study,' [22].

There is the fear that women who stop wearing bras after reading *'Dressed to Kill'* will also stop engaging in breast screening programmes believing that the mammograms may be doing more harm than good if their risk of breast cancer is believed to be inherently very low.

I will first summarise and discuss the results of the *'Dressed To Kill'* questionnaire, then examine the pressure exerted by your bra on the lymphatic system.

The Singer and Grismaijer Questionnaire

Singer and Grismaijer argue that bra-wearing may be a major cause of breast cancer. The authors claim that breast cancer is only a problem in cultures where women wear bras; in bra-free cultures, breast cancer is a rare event.

Singer and Grismaijer noticed that the Maori of New Zealand, who are integrated into white culture and therefore mostly wear bras, have the same rate of breast cancer as the Caucasian New Zealanders. Breast cancer is virtually unknown in bra-free Maoris.

Also the aboriginals of Australia, who are bra-free, have almost no breast cancer. The same polarisation is true for 'Westernized' Japanese, Fijians and other bra-converted cultures where breast cancer rates increase to the levels endemic in the population into which they assimilate whilst their bra-free compatriots are essentially free of cancer.

Whatever the causes of breast cancer there are large differences in incidence rates around the world [23].

Might not the increased risk of breast cancer be more likely due to the change to a western diet, being overweight, being exposed to toxins and pollution, etc., which are conventionally believed to be the causes of the disease than simply wearing a bra?

Singer and Grismaijer examined the bra wearing statistics of over 4,700 US women in five major cities. They claim about half of the women questioned had had breast cancer.

The proportion of all women who suffer breast cancer is significantly less than half of the population so women with breast cancer have either been deliberately encouraged to join the survey or women breast cancer sufferers have pro-actively joined the survey.

This has been a cause for concern from critics of the survey.

Those taking part should not be aware of the aims of any survey otherwise the attitudes of the volunteers and their responses may well be skewed to a point of being invalid. Women with breast cancer will naturally be very anxious to make a contribution to uncovering the causes of the disease and finding a universal cure. This will usually bias results.

It was also strongly argued that correlations found from the survey do not necessarily indicate a causal relationship as I will now demonstrate.

A false correlation?

The authors of *'Dressed to Kill'* claimed that 3 out of 4 women who wore their bras 24 hours per day developed breast cancer and that 1 out of 7 women who wore bras more than 12 hour per day but not to bed developed breast cancer.

In addition, 1 out of 152 women who wore their bras less than 12 hours per day got breast cancer and 1 out of 168 women who wore bras rarely or never suffered breast cancer. Their study also claims that bra-free women have about the same incidence of breast cancer as men.

This appears at first sight to be very powerful evidence that bra wearing causes cancer.

DOES BRA WEARING CREATE HEALTH PROBLEMS?

There is an established relationship between Body Mass Index (BMI) [24] and incidence of breast cancer at least in pre-menopausal women [25].

There is also a well established relationship between BMI and breast size [26].

Being generally overweight after the menopause is linked with an increased risk of breast cancer. Oestrogen can encourage the growth of breast cancer and after the menopause your oestrogen levels are linked to how much fat you have.

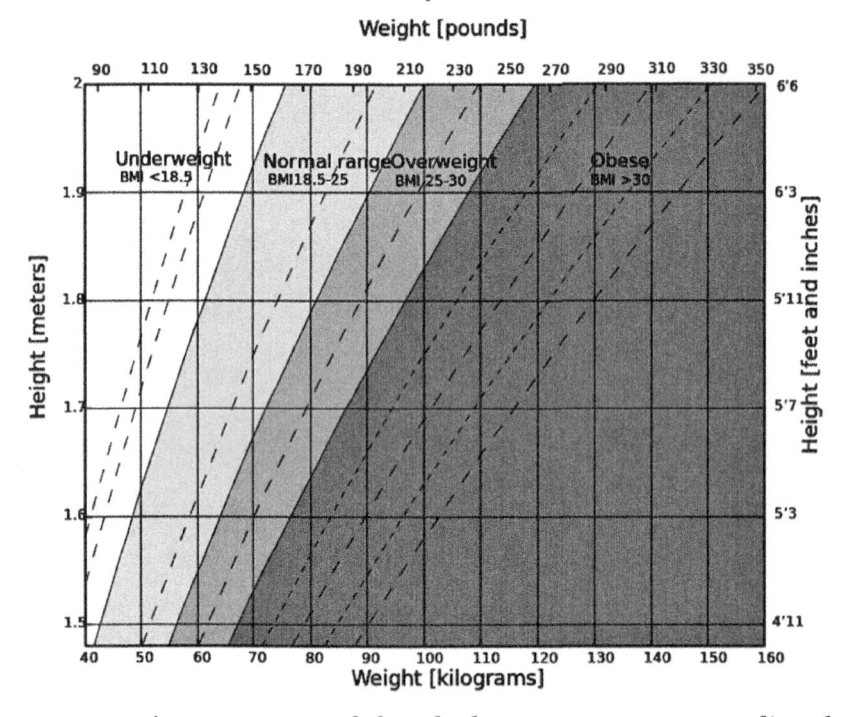

In 2010, nine per cent of female breast cancers were directly linked to women being overweight or obese ten years earlier [27].

In addition, for the smaller bodied woman with a Body Mass Index (BMI) below 25 kg/m², those with a bra cup size of 'D or larger' had a significantly higher incidence of breast cancer than women who reported 'A or smaller' cup size.

Larger bra cup size at a young age is associated with a higher incidence of premenopausal breast cancer [28].

Women with large BMIs tend to wear larger sized bras which probably are worn for longer hours each day than smaller women

DOES BRA WEARING CREATE HEALTH PROBLEMS?

do.

Women with obese BMI values above 30 kg/m² will predominantly have very large breasts and may well wear bras all day and night for comfort. They also have the highest risk of breast cancer because of their obesity and probable poor life style and diet.

Very slender women with small or no perceptible breasts might rarely, if ever, wear bras and they are also the women least likely to contract breast cancer.

For example, we can read that women with a C cup have four times the risk of breast cancer death compared to those with an A cup. Those with a D cup or larger had nearly five times the risk of the A-cup women [29].

This same research paper shows a strong relationship between exercise levels and fitness and breast cancer risk.

So, could it not be true that larger breasted women will wear their bras for longer each day and even all night and take less exercise?

Isn't it a fact that older women are more likely than their younger generations to wear bras longer each day out of long-term habit and breast cancer risks increase with age particularly post-menopause?

So, we have the observation that the two groups of women - high BMI and post-menopausal - that have elevated risks of breast cancer are also the same women that are likely to wear bras for longer each day.

In which case, how can the medical professionals blame age and weight rather than bra wearing habits for breast cancer enhanced risk?

Have any studies been conducted relating breast cancer risks to age, weight AND bra wearing habits so that the effect of the three variables can be untangled?

This does not appear to have been studied in the 'Dressed to Kill' survey.

Singer and Grismaijer admit that the strict protocols necessary to unravel the individual effects of possible breast cancer risk enhancing parameters like those just demonstrated were not followed. This was because the authors hoped that the medical industry would conduct follow-up studies to either verify or refute their findings.

The book *'Dressed to Kill'* generated controversy - hardly surprising! The authors attributed the greed of the fashion and medical industries to the lack of follow-up studies and the perceived casual dismissal of their conclusions.

The authors claim that the mainstream medical organizations all denied the link between smoking and lung cancer for decades after the initial research was published and they make the same accusation against the bra industry.

This is rather unfair because the rubbishing of claims linking tobacco smoking to lung cancer were systematically financed and orchestrated by the tobacco industry and opposed by the medical profession.

There is little reason to think that the bra industry could suppress a link between bra wearing and breast cancer by persuading, threatening and bribing countless oncologists, researchers and doctors to join in this 'conspiracy'. In these days of social media, whistleblowing and investigative journalism such a conspiracy would be either unthinkable or profoundly stupid.

In my view the situation is more closely related to the extraordinary story of the discovery of the true cause of stomach ulcers.

Back in the 1950s John Lykoudis, a general practitioner in Greece, treated patients for peptic ulcer disease with antibiotics long before it was commonly recognized that bacteria were a dominant cause for the disease. [30]

Helicobacter pylori were rediscovered in 1982 by two Australian scientists, Robin Warren and Barry J. Marshall as a causative factor for ulcers.

In their original paper, Warren and Marshall contended that most gastric ulcers and gastritis were caused by colonization with this bacterium, not by stress or spicy food as had been assumed until then.

In 1972 I developed a stomach ulcer and was treated with antacid tablets, which suppressed the symptoms, and anti-stress pills despite the fact that I had no stress in my life apart from the birth of my first child which was far more pleasurable than stressful!

DOES BRA WEARING CREATE HEALTH PROBLEMS?

The hypothesis that Helicobacter pylori were the cause of stomach ulcers was poorly received.

So Marshall drank from a Petri dish containing a culture of organisms extracted from a patient with gastritis and five days later developed gastritis. This experiment was published in 1984 in the Australian Medical Journal and is among the most cited articles from the journal.

In 1986, Dr Barry Marshall was invited to discuss it at a gastroenterology conference in the United States. His wife came along and, while doing some sightseeing, overheard a conversation among some other gastroenterologists' wives who happened to be sitting in front of her on a bus. They referred to *'...this terrible person that they imported from Australia to speak,'* and went on *'How could they put such rubbish in the conference?'* [31]

However, it was not until 1997 that a national education campaign to inform health care providers and consumers about the link between Helicobacter pylori and ulcers was started in the UK.

In 2005, Marshall and his long-time collaborator Dr. Warren were awarded the Nobel Prize in Physiology or Medicine *'for their discovery of the bacterium Helicobacter pylori and its role in gastritis and peptic ulcer disease.'*

I have told this tale to show that scientists can be stubborn and make mistakes and that progress can be very slow. However, scientists are not (or at least very rarely) evil. They would not rubbish the book *'Dressed to Kill'* because of pressure from the bra industry in order that a possible cure for breast cancer could be suppressed for financial gain. Such a claim would be grotesque.

'Dressed to Kill' - A Selection of Questionnaire Results

Returning to the questionnaire answers and leaving conspiracy theories behind us, I found that most of the results are curious and worthy of note.

The following are a selection of questions and answers.

'Are you comfortable with the size and shape of your breasts without a bra?'

Non-cancer group 18% Yes, Cancer group 5% Yes.

The authors believe that this polarisation of dissatisfaction arises from the perception of breasts by men in male dominated societies and women's need to conform to this template.

This is probably correct although, as we saw on earlier, to be flat chested was to be desirable in the 1920s.

What I found intriguing was the poor self-assessment of their breasts by typical breast cancer sufferers.

Is this a clue to the apparent correlation between cancer and breast self-perception or is it just a false memory created by cancer sufferers looking back and feeling that they have cancer because their bra choices were bad?

This is where the lack of a strict protocol shows potential weaknesses in the conclusions. The volunteers answering the survey questions must have realised that the survey was about the relationship between bra wearing and breast cancer and this would have influenced their answers.

It is for this reason that trials and survey need to be 'double blind' to avoid bias.

'Do you select bras to shape or accentuate your breasts?'

Non-cancer group 74% Yes, Cancer group 87% Yes.

Nothing very contentious here. It shows that the majority of women in the USA consider bras to be an important feature of their appearance.

'Apart from price what is the most important feature you look for when buying a bra?'

Non-cancer group 30% Appearance, 51% Comfort and 19% Both

Cancer group 62% Appearance, 25%, Comfort and 13% Both

The cancer group of women put twice as much emphasis on appearance as the non-cancer group.

I found this remarkable and revealing.

Could it be that choosing a bra to enhance appearance at the expense of comfort is correlated in some way with the chance of developing breast cancer?

Could this result be biased in any way by the way the survey was setup?

Is the fact that many women may have been disproportionately selected to take part because they have breast cancer thereby

DOES BRA WEARING CREATE HEALTH PROBLEMS?

influencing the answer to that question?

Could women with breast cancer be retrospectively blaming their lifestyle choice in bra buying for their illness and be distorting their recollection of their bra buying motives?

'Does your bra occasionally feel tight or uncomfortable?'

Non-cancer group 28% Rarely, 55% Sometimes and 17% Always

Cancer group 48% Rarely, 34%, Sometimes and 18% Always

Clearly there is no significant difference between the cancer group and non-cancer group when it comes to wearing bras that always feel tight and uncomfortable. This implies that wearing badly fitting bras does not correlate with breast cancer problems.

However, where the clear distinction comes is where we see that women who rarely find their bras uncomfortable are about twice as likely to succumb to breast cancer as those whose bras are rarely uncomfortable and tight.

This appears to go against the hypothesis that tight and uncomfortable bras are linked with breast cancer.

'Does your bra ever make red marks on your skin or cause irritation?'

Non-cancer group 25% Rarely, 52% Sometimes and 23% Always

Cancer group 14% Rarely, 46%, Sometimes and 40% Always

Sydney Ross Singer and Soma Grismaijer took these results to demonstrate that bras so ill-fitting and uncomfortable that they left red marks were implicated in breast cancer.

The book authors discuss this paradox at length and broadly conclude that women who regard bras as essential items to ensure attractive appearance are less likely to complain about a bra that leaves red marks. These women treat discomfort as a 'necessary evil' and don't always report an attractive bra as uncomfortable.

'How long do you wear your bra each day on the average?'

Non-cancer group: 20% less than 12 hours daily

Cancer group: 1% less than 12 hours.

The authors discuss this result for four pages but the clear result shouts out that bra wearing more than 12 hours a day correlates

DOES BRA WEARING CREATE HEALTH PROBLEMS?

with breast cancer increase.

However, cause and effect can be very different.

Would not a larger woman with an 'overweight' BMI find comfort from having more hours of bra support than a slender woman?

Medical experience is that increasing BMI and bra cup sizes increase the risk of breast cancer.

'Do you wear your bra or breast supporting garment to sleep?'

Non-cancer group: 3% yes

Cancer group: 18% yes

There are other questions, answers and discussions in the book 'Dressed to Kill' and it is well worth reading all the answers and the deductions.

The following table summarises the results from the 'Dress to Kill' survey and is based on a chart in the book.

Remember that the bra wearing regime is supposed to be the one used before the breast cancer was diagnosed.

	Cancer Group	Non-Cancer Group
Bra is not worn	0.24%	5%
Bra is worn less than 12 hours each day.	1%	19%
Bra is worn more than 12 hours each day but not to sleep in.	81%	73%
Bra is worn all the time	18%	3%

Throughout the discussion of the results of the questionnaire the authors pursue their hypothesis that wearing bras interferes with the lymphatic drainage system and results in toxins accumulating in the breasts thereby increasing the risk of breast cancer.

It is true that cancer victims did tend, before their illness struck, to wear bras longer each day, wear bras in bed and report red pressure marks more often. However, without taking into account the bra wearing habits of women as a function of age and BMI no conclusions can be drawn about the influence of bra wearing on

DOES BRA WEARING CREATE HEALTH PROBLEMS?

breast cancer risk.

I am not saying that bra wearing might not be a contributing factor towards the incidence of breast cancer. I am simply saying that the evidence from the questionnaire is inconclusive because the correct protocols have not been carried out as pointed out by numerous cancer and general health experts.

What is difficult to explain is the extraordinarily strong correlation between hours per day of bra wearing and breast cancer susceptibility.

Can the medical fraternity explain how being bra free correlates so strongly with very low breast cancer incidence unless the triggers, such as genetics, obesity, smoking, diet, pre- and post-menopause, etc., actually have very little influence?

Can so much expensive research have been wrong in teasing out these contributing factors when it was just bra wearing all along that is the problem?

As stated earlier, Singer and Grismaijer did not have the resources to conduct a survey that would satisfy the most pedantic scientist - and there are a lot of them out there! I know because I worked as a professional scientist for 45 years - both employed and freelance - and I've met all types of pedants.

What is urgently needed is a properly resourced and conducted survey to settle the issue of whether bra wearing does increase the risk of contracting breast cancer.

With over 450,000 women dying worldwide every year from breast cancer [32] why has this not been done?

It can hardly have been through lack of money with the US Government talking of spending as much as $150 billion to send a few humans to Mars (for what purpose?) and spending $9 billion launching the James Webb Telescope into space [33] to examine minute details about how the universe formed - a topic of no conceivable value to the lives and health of us humans who pay the bills.

I will end this section with a chart showing the incidence of breast cancer in various countries plotted against the Gross Domestic Product (GDP) per head of the population.

DOES BRA WEARING CREATE HEALTH PROBLEMS?

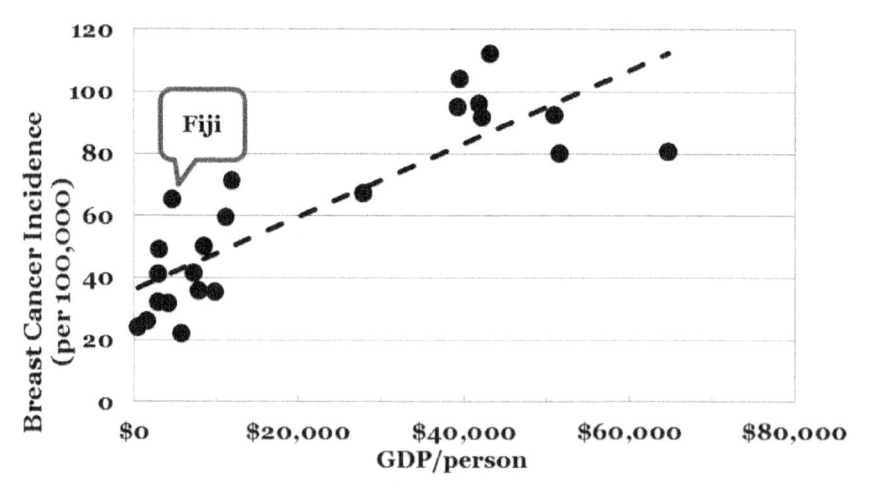

The countries represented on this chart range from the richest (USA, Sweden, Canada) to the poorest (Niger, Vanuatu, Egypt).

It can be seen that there is a clear relationship between breast cancer incidence and the wealth (and hence lifestyle) of countries.

Fiji is indicated because Singer and Grismaijer have used this island nation to show that women who wear bras appear to have a much greater incidence of breast cancer than women who remain traditionally bra-less.

Some of the countries plotted in the lower left corner of the chart (the poorest nations) are traditionally bra wearing whilst others are traditionally bra-less.

It is clear to me that, even in the poorest countries, the breast cancer rates are never zero and are never lower than about one-third of the rates in the richest countries.

The 'lymphatic blockage' theory of breast cancer suggests that there should be data points much lower than an incidence rate of 20 per 100,000 for non-bra wearing countries.

To me this chart supports the traditional hypothesis that lifestyle- is a major factor in breast cancer risk and not bra wearing.

Others will no doubt disagree.

Under Pressure.

The arguments about the effects of a bra on breast function and specifically the operation of the lymphatic system revolves around pressure. A breast is under pressure at all times.

DOES BRA WEARING CREATE HEALTH PROBLEMS?

When bra-free the breast behaves like a bag of fluid suspended from the ribcage.

OK!

That's really a big turn-off for all those who enjoy breasts in so many ways. But, looking at a breast as a bag of fluid allows us to understand the stresses and strains that they have to cope with both when stationary and when jiggling during a workout at the gym.

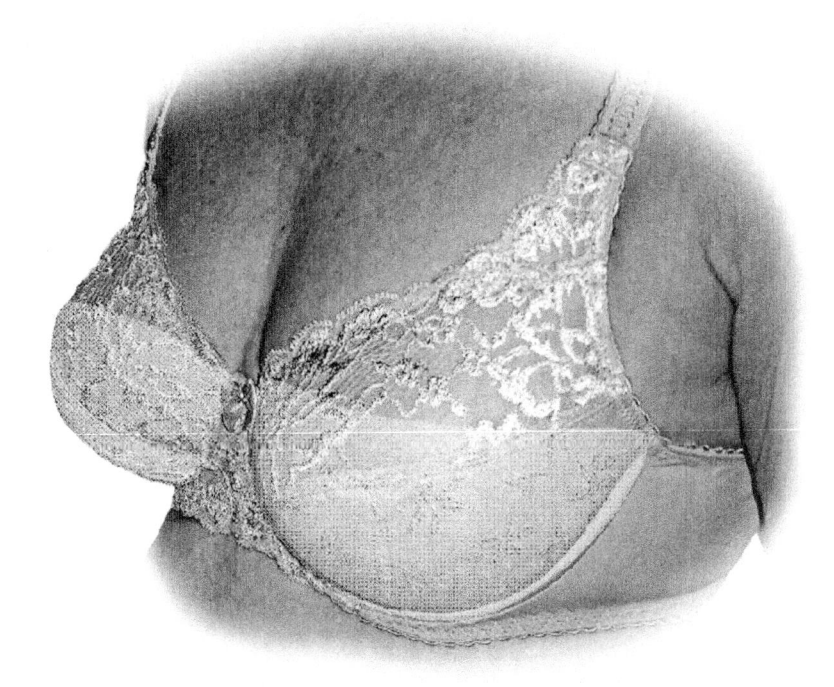

First let's remember that 80% of the weight of each breast is carried by the bottom part of the bra cup as shown by the shaded area in the above picture.

The average pressure exerted on the breasts by the bra cup is equal to about 80% of the weight of the breast distributed over the area of the bra cup shaded.

As a result of measuring the bra cup areas of the many bras in my collection and knowing the weight of a breast [34] we can easily find the average pressure exerted by the cups as shown in the table below for typical bra sizes.

DOES BRA WEARING CREATE HEALTH PROBLEMS?

UK Bra Size	US Bra Size	Cup Pressure (pascals)
32A	32AA	571
34E	34DD/E	1,099
38D	38C	1,121
42DD	42D	1,483
42G	42H	1,860

Hang on - what's this 'pascal' we have encountered? It is the metric (SI) unit of pressure. It is named after Blaise Pascal - shown below - one of the founders of the mathematical theory of chance and probability [35].

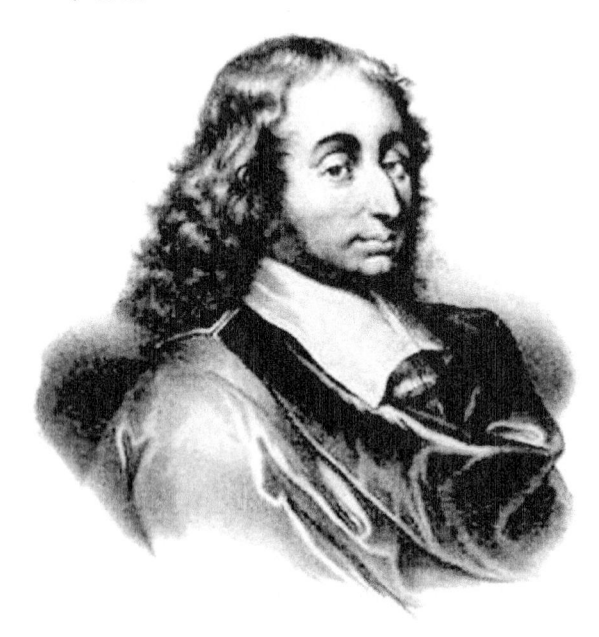

When a gambler friend asked if he could work out (for example) the chance of throwing a double six with two dice he sat down and invented probability theory. Thanks to Blaise, his friend made a fortune at the gaming tables and Pascal effectively invented Las

DOES BRA WEARING CREATE HEALTH PROBLEMS?

Vegas.

The pressure of a full bottle of wine standing on the palm of your hand is about 3,200 pascals. That's about double the pressure that your breasts are experiencing from your bra cups.

Looking back at the table above we see that the pressure of a bra cup pressing on the breast is really quite high when imagined in terms of that wine bottle pressing down on your hand.

Having stayed with this little book thus far you deserve a large glass - go on! Pour it and enjoy!

There is another way to estimate the pressure on and within a breast.

Visualise a breast as a bag of fluid contained by the skin which is under stress. The pressure at the lowest point of the breast differs from the pressure at the top by about 1,200 pascals because the breast tissue at the bottom of the breast is being pressed upon by the tissue above.

Yet another calculation I have made is of the pressure of the bra band on the ribcage under the armpit which is where the bra band pressure is greatest.

I won't bore you with the details of how I calculated this underarm pressure except to say that it involved stretching many bras and measuring the force needed to clip a bra around a ribcage.

This was done by suspending bras from their hooks and hanging weights onto the eyes. Various weights were used to find the force as a function of extension.

By measuring the stretching needed to do up the hooks and eyes on the bra for a given ribcage size and by measuring the area of the bra band I was able to work out the tension in a bra band and then to calculate the pressure the band exerts on the underarm ribcage.

DOES BRA WEARING CREATE HEALTH PROBLEMS?

Here are a few values calculated for typical bra sizes.

UK Bra Size	US Bra Size	Underarm Pressure (Pascals)
30AA	30AAA	2,156
32A	32AA	1,730
34D	34C	1,380
36B	36A	1,899
40D	40C	1,970
42E	42DD	1,744

It can be seen that the underarm pressure is between about 1,400 and 2,200 pascals averaged over the bra band under the arm.

Most bra bands have a fairly stiff edging and the pressure can be concentrated in this thin strip of fabric. In this case the pressure may be significantly higher over a narrow strip around the edge of the bra band than shown in the above table.

This is where the bra leaves unhealthy red marks.

At this point I must pay tribute to my longsuffering partner who watched some of her favourite bras being stretched and tortured beyond their normal extent.

The pressure exerted by a bra has been directly measured by David Moth who carried out a remarkable experiment measuring the pressure at various points of his wife's bra where it presses on her ribcage [36].

It is worth nothing that Marks & Spenser has a remarkable innovation when it comes to fitting bras. It has a device to measure the pressure between the bra and the skin. [64]

DOES BRA WEARING CREATE HEALTH PROBLEMS?

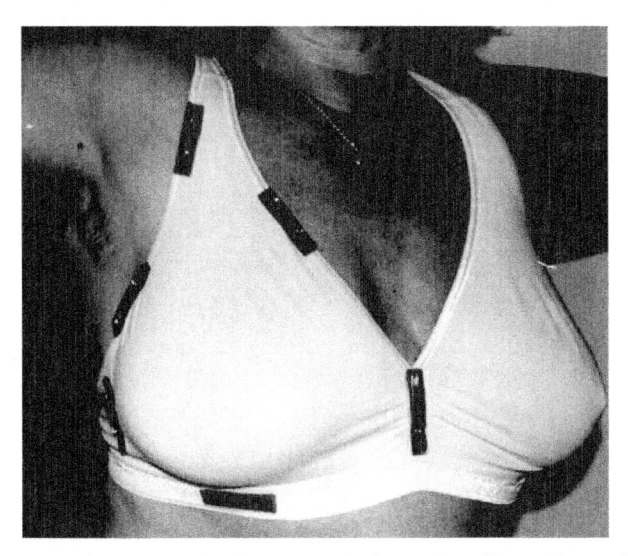

The above picture (which David has kindly allowed me to reproduce) shows transducer attachments at various places on a bra.

The following table shows the pressures measured.

Position	Pressure (pascals)
Front Shoulder Strap	1,250
Mid-underarm	2,500
Inner Edge Cup	3,750
Back Shoulder Strap	4,375
Mid Chest	6,250
Mid Upper Back Strap	6,250
Outer Edge Cup	8,750
Back Underbust	11,250
Front Underbust	11,870
Mid Back Strap	13,100
Lower Back Strap	14,380
Shoulder strap	16,900

DOES BRA WEARING CREATE HEALTH PROBLEMS?

It can be seen that the measured pressures are substantial and highly variable from point to point on the bra.

Of particular note is that David's measurement under the armpit is 2,500 pascals and this is comparable to the predictions of 1,380 to 2,156 pascals made by my theory of bra pressure bearing in mind that I have been predicting the average pressure exerted by the bra band whereas David has measured the more localised pressure of the edge of the bra band.

It's time to think about five full bottles of wine balancing on top of each other sitting on the palm of your hand. The pressure on your hand is the pressure on David's wife's bra strap!

So, we have seen that pressure on the breasts and ribcage can vary over a wide range for different sizes of bras and these pressures are large.

What effect can these pressures have on your comfort and health?

Frankly, there is no way to say because the research has not been done as far as I can find.

However, we do know a little about the pressures involved in the lymphatic system which drains lymph fluids from the breasts [37]. Twelve patients with primary and secondary lymphedema were studied before treatment, after two weeks of intensive physical therapy and three months of continuing compression and ergotherapy.

After two weeks of intensive manual lymph drainage and compression bandaging microlymphatic hypertension was down from 1,700 pascals to a mean lymph capillary pressure of 800 pascals.

More than three months later after continuing compression a lymph capillary pressure of 425 pascals was reported.

So we see that the healthy lymphatic pressure is about 400 - 800 pascals which is significantly lower than the pressure exerted by the bra on the breasts and the ribcage.

Is this a problem?

I don't know and I'm not qualified to speculate. I am just a septuagenarian pensioner with no medical training but with an interest in improving women's health.

Many readers seeing these pressure figures would be sure that the lymphatic drainage system would be interrupted by such external pressures well in excess of the pressures in the system.

Consider the analogy of a hosepipe buried under ground. It is subject to high pressures from the soil above and around it but it will not collapse if the pipe walls are sufficiently rigid to keep their shape. Water will still flow unimpeded if the pipe walls are sufficiently strong.

How rigid are the minute pipes through which lymph fluid flows?

It appears that nobody knows.

However, the pressure in a bra-free breast is about 1,200 pascals different from top to bottom simply due to the support provided by the ligaments and this pressure is three times the healthy lymphatic pressure of about 400 pascals.

If a breast *au naturel* can operate perfectly well with internal pressures several times greater than the lymphatic pressure how can any opinion be given as to the ability of the lymphatic system to operate with the higher pressures imposed by wearing a bra?

Even if wearing a bra in the day does interfere with the lymphatic system, does taking off a bra at night allow the lymphatic system to operate and do its job satisfactorily?

Here again I am not qualified to comment and nobody appears to have investigated this question.

Perhaps the most difficult evidence for Singer and Grismaijer to counter is the statement that many women have had their breast lymph nodes removed for non-cancer related health issues and yet these women have shown no increase in breast cancer risk.

Dr. Gansler and colleagues compared National Cancer Institute data on breast cancer risk for women treated for melanoma who had several underarm lymph nodes removed and those who did not. The surgery, which is known to block lymph drainage from breast tissue, did not detectably increase breast cancer rates, the study found, meaning that it is extremely unlikely that wearing a bra, which affects lymph flow, would do so.

However, Singer countered this assertion on his blog in a post dated 10 October 2013 [38]

Sydney Singer also cites references to support his hypothesis. For example a 1991 Harvard study [39] found that, premenopausal women who do not wear bras had half the risk of breast cancer compared with bra users.

However, the authors stated that this link was likely to be due to factors related to wearing a bra rather than the bra itself. The women in the study who did not wear a bra were more likely to be lean, which the authors concluded might account for the lower risk [40].

In addition, Singer and Grismaijer did a follow-up study in Fiji. They found 24 case histories of breast cancer in a culture where half the women are bra-free. The women getting breast cancer were all wearing bras. Given women with the same genetics and diet and living in the same village, the ones getting breast disease were the ones wearing bras for work [41].

A 2009 Chinese study found that not sleeping in a bra was protective against breast cancer, lowering the risk 60%. [42]

In 2011 a study was published in Spanish confirming that bras are causing breast disease and cancer. It found that underwired and push-up bras are the most harmful, but any bra that leaves red marks or indentations may cause disease. [43]

In summary, I cannot give any opinion on the claims that bra wearing can be a factor in causing breast cancer.

Until a large enough survey is carried out into this claim which addresses all the epidemiology requirements and protocols, the claim by Singer and Grismaijer that bra wearing may be a contributing cause of breast cancer cannot be proved or disproved.

With over 450,000 women dying worldwide every year from breast cancer [44] why has this urgently needed study not been done?

Get It Off!

In 2000 Singer and Grismaijer published a book reiterating the conclusions of 'Dressed To Kill' [45]. A little more information was included. However, this did not substantially add to the material in their previous book.

Curiously this second book is largely taken up by an 'opera' being an enactment of the evils of bra wearing.

Whilst amusing as a way of illustrating the perceived evils of bra wearing and indoctrination of women into buying bras as sex garments, this book does not significantly push forward the authors' thesis that blockage of the lymphatic system is the cause of breast cancer in bra wearing women.

The book does recommend that woman try leaving their bras off for a month or so to see how it feels. Although this is far too short a time to have noticeable effects on breast cancer vulnerability there may be a significant beneficial effect on breast pain which would be well worth trying.

The Singer and Grismaijer blog is well worth following [46].

'Bras: The Bare Facts'

On 2nd November 2000 the UK TV Channel 4 broadcast an investigation into the health risks of bras and bra wearing habits.

There is a transcript of this TV documentary available [47].

The programme started with some chilling facts.

In the UK 2 out of 5 women suffer pains in their breasts and 1 in 7 suffers cysts.

Breast cancer rates in the Developed World were 1 in 20 sufferers in 1900 rising to 1 in 10 by 1970. (By 2010 the rate was 1 in 3 sufferers.)

Reference was made by the researchers to a French study which stated that breast pain was a strong risk of breast cancer and as great a risk as family history.

Channel 4 sponsored a six month study conducted at the Frenchay Hospital, Bristol UK by Dr Simon Cawthorn of Frenchay Hospital and Dr Robert Mansel of University College of Wales at Cardiff.

Dr Cawthorn stated that women buy bras for appearance and not comfort whilst Dr Mansel stated

"There is no positive evidence of bras being good for breasts. Where bras are not worn there is no breast cancer."

Dr Marlene Schuytvlot who was Registrar at the Frenchay Hospital in 2000 stated that

"85% of lymph nodes in breasts drain to the armpit. All the lymphatic flow comes to a region where the edge of the bra presses on the skin. This could restrict flow and might lead to breast problems."

DOES BRA WEARING CREATE HEALTH PROBLEMS?

One hundred women attending a 'Breast Pain Clinic' at the Frenchay Hospital in Bristol volunteered to join in a research study. The volunteers were asked to wear their normal bras for three months and then to go without a bra for three months.

At the start of the experiment all the women suffered breast pain and most had benign cysts at the start of the study.

Some quotes from the programme include the following:

Rae Marsh, a volunteer in the study, stated that her breast pain was so great that she could not pick up her children.

'Breast pain is a major problem for 60% - 70% of women.'

'Sufferers of pain and cysts fear cancer'

'I have to hold my breasts sometimes due to the pain. There is a continual ache.'

'As far as cysts and breast pain are concerned facts are very sparse.'

'My doctor has recommended wearing firm bras to help with my breast pain and cysts'

In fact the outcome of the study was the opposite advice!

The main result of the study was a 7% increase in pain-free days for pre-menopausal women whilst not wearing a bra

For women suffering 'moderate' or 'severe' breast pain the number of days with such pain was halved.

This was considered to be highly significant.

No influence was found on the rate of production of cysts or on the lifetime of cysts.

Because cysts may develop into breast cancer it was concluded that bra wearing does not increase the risk of breast cancer, at least through the mechanism of creating and developing cysts.

Individuals taking part in the study had mixed reactions as shown by the following quotes by participants.

'My cysts improved but I went back to wearing a bra out of habit. It's important to be the same as everyone else. I conform. I don't want to be thought of as that woman who doesn't wear a bra.'

'You don't think that a bra can be causing the pain because they

DOES BRA WEARING CREATE HEALTH PROBLEMS?

are advertised for comfort, control and support.'

'I feel nicer without my bras. I've got rid of them.'

'I've been given back my freedom. Breast pain has gone, my worry has stopped and I'm enjoying life more.'

'The trial was magic! I'll never go back to wearing a bra.'

The reason some women returned to bra wearing despite the reduction in breast pain was because they were afraid their nipples would show. Some women who left off their bras wore shirts with pockets to hide their nipples. Other were afraid of unwanted nipple erections due to the sensitively of the nipple and aureole to friction with clothing.

If this worries you then Google 'nipple covers' to buy flesh coloured self-adhesive covers and you can watch George Clooney at the pictures without your nipples displaying your true feelings for him!

In the US there is a brand of nipple covers called 'Dimrs' - because they solve the head light problem!

The Frenchay researchers stated that they would follow up this research with further studies but I have found no reports of any additional work.

No further studies investigating a possible relationship between bra wearing and breast pain has been carried out as far as I can discover.

John Dixey the General Manager of Playtex dismissed criticism of bra wearing and possible related health issues saying that

'Playtex will not sponsor research into health issues but will listen to the results.'

He dismissed criticism of bra wearing as *'Hearsay from non-medical commentators'*.

However, Professor Jean-Christophe Thalabard, University of Paris Hospital said

'The reason why we were astonished by the results (is) the fact that usually when we look at some risk factor for breast cancer, the order of magnitude is 1.1 or 1.2. It's not so high, I mean.

When you go to 2 and above (double the risk, which is what they found for breast pain), it usually deals with familial factors,

DOES BRA WEARING CREATE HEALTH PROBLEMS?

personal history of breast disease, but not for ... common clinical symptoms. So it was for us something which was astonishingly high.'

'I would say that reducing breast pain is an objective by itself, because you need to have a normal life without pain. And if it turns out that it is really connected with a reduction of breast cancer, it might be very important from a public health point of view."

In this TV programme Professor Hugh Simpson measured the increase in temperature of breasts caused by bra wearing. He found an increase of about 0.5 degrees Centigrade.

Although not a large amount, any increase in tissue temperature can indicate an increase in the risk of breast cancer. When screening women for pre-cancerous symptoms a temperature rise of just 0.5 degree is taken as an indicator of the need for further investigation.

We must be very careful here not to draw a false conclusion.

A natural increase of 0.5 degree in breast temperature may be an indicator of a pre-cancerous breast condition but that does not mean that artificially raising the temperature of a breast by the same amount by wearing a bra increases the risk of breast cancer.

A false comparison has been made with the observed drop in sperm production when testicles are warmed by the wearing of tight underwear. This is unrelated to cancer of the testicles but rather a natural reaction to testicles being warmed to an unnatural level which causes sperm production rate to fall.

Simon Cawthorn, Consultant Surgeon at the Frenchay Hospital stated in the TV programme

'It is possible that a cooler breast is a healthier breast'

This TV programme was widely - and generally erroneously - reported in the UK newspapers as showing that bra wearing increased the risk of breast cancer. [48]

It did not. The main results of the study was a 7% increase in pain-free days for pre-menopausal women whilst not wearing a bra and a halving of the number of days when the breast pain was rated 'Moderate' or 'Severe'.

This is a very significant result but falls short of proving that bra

DOES BRA WEARING CREATE HEALTH PROBLEMS?

wearing causes breast cancer.

The responses of representatives of various cancer organisations were intriguing and sometimes disappointing [49].

For example, a representative of the 'Cancer Research Organisation' was reported as saying

'There is no substantiated evidence to link wearing a bra to breast cancer and I am very worried that women will be unnecessarily worried by this suggestion.'

A spokeswoman for the 'Breast Cancer Care' charity stated

'The findings (of this study) need to be treated with caution and not reported out of proportion since most women in the UK wear a bra and this could cause considerable alarm.'

A 'Breakthrough Breast Cancer' representative said

'There is no scientific evidence to suggest that wearing a well-fitting bra causes breast pain or breast cancer. A good-fitting bra supports the ligaments in the breasts to prevent them from overstretching. Women should be properly measured for their bras and they should be tried on to ensure a good fit."

There are two errors in this statement. The Frenchay Hospital study did indeed show that bra wearing correlates with breast pain intensity and wearing a bra is known to make sagging worse not better.

A spokesman from the 'Imperial Cancer Research Fund' stated:

'It is a very small study which focuses on breast pain. The results suggest that there might be an effect, but it's far too early to establish a definite connection between bras and breast pain.'

How much more evidence is needed before the medical professionals will admit even to the smallest possibility of a relationship between bra wearing and breast health?

Recent Progress

A thorough search of websites, medical research papers and books has failed to turn up any significant progress in the study of the relationship between wearing bras and breast health.

There is much anecdotal information such as the following from 2011.

DOES BRA WEARING CREATE HEALTH PROBLEMS?

'I have suffered from fibrocystic breasts my entire adult life. At age 52, the lumps in my breasts had become so numerous, large and painful I could no longer ignore them.

After doing some research online, I stopped wearing a bra. After about a week the pain and tenderness disappeared and now, four months later, the lumps have all gone away with none taking their place. This result has been dramatic and transformational for me. I wanted to share it with other women since this is a very common condition.

Needless to say, this treatment costs nothing and has no side effects. I wish my doctor had told me about this.' [50]

This shows how little progress has been made over the past decade investigating women's breast health and its relationship with bra wearing and how little of what has been know for decades has reached the bra wearing women of our world.

Summary

There is no overall conclusion that can be reached here.

The survey by Singer and Grismaijer shows a strong correlation between bra wearing and breast cancer. In particular, the more hours each days a bra is worn the higher the incidence of breast cancer.

However, there is no way of knowing which way this correlation applies. Does bra wearing cause cancer directly or do women who habitually wear bras for many hours each day have a lifestyle (smoking, drinking alcohol, being overweight, number of pregnancies, etc.) that increases their chance of getting breast cancer?

Singer and Grismaijer state that Fijian women who don't wear bras have no breast cancer but those who change to a Westernised lifestyle do get breast cancer. Could this be due to the lifestyle change of which bra wearing is a part?

If a significant proportion of Fijian women still go bra-less then why does Fiji have a breast cancer incidence rate higher than found in countries with similar lifestyles and economies as shown by the earlier chart.

I have raised the possibility in this chapter that the correlation found by Singer and Grismaijer was due to the likelihood that heavier women who are known to be more susceptible to breast cancer have heavier breasts and wear their bras for more hours each day.

Maybe the Singer and Grismaijer effect is a reflection of the Body Mass Index of the women and lifestyle rather than the bra wearing habits.

I have also raised the reverse possibility that studies which show an increase in breast cancer risk with body weight might actually be observing the effect of wearing bras for more hours each day which would vindicate Singer and Grismaijer.

Despite the protestations by the medical profession and bra manufacturers that there is no evidence linking bra wearing and breast cancer, there are studies by French, Japanese, Chinese and Spanish researchers that show significant correlations supporting the Singer and Grismaijer survey.

When a professional scientist dismisses an observation that he or she does not like the response is often *'There is no published evidence to support that observation!'*

It is one of the fundamental rules of science that

'Absence of evidence is not evidence of absence'

If contrary evidence does not exist it is usually because nobody has looked for it. A presumed absence of evidence to support the work of Singer and Grismaijer means nothing more than nobody has done the research to follow up on their pioneering work.

The theory that breast cancer could be induced by the pressure of a bra cutting off the flow of lymphatic fluids is unproven but is plausible. It is supported by experts such as Dr Marlene Schuytvlot who was Registrar of the Frenchay Hospital in 2000.

The claim that removing the lymph nodes in women's breast does not increase susceptibility to cancer appears to refute the Singer and Grismaijer hypothesis that lymph blockage is the link between bra wearing and breast cancer. However Singer and Grismaijer dismiss the contrary evidence as not peer reviewed research - exactly the same argument used against their own work!

Touché!

Frankly, the evidence for and against the lymph node blockage hypothesis simply isn't strong enough to make a judgement.

The Frenchay Hospital study showed that not wearing a bra gave

DOES BRA WEARING CREATE HEALTH PROBLEMS?

relief to many women suffering from cysts and breast pain. However, these conditions do not necessarily lead to breast cancer.

If there is a single statement that sums up this chapter it is that research into breast cancer and the possible effects of bra wearing have been tragically under investigated and that the resources applied to this topic have been pathetic.

One feature running through this chapter is that women have been relentlessly manipulated by the massive bra industry into believing that bras are essential tools for ensnaring a mate. This is a post-1940s phenomenon driven by ruthless advertising of which the 'Hello Boys' Wonderbra advertisement was the most iconic and disgraceful in recent decades [51], [52].

Given that women are - sadly - unlikely to go through another 1960s type of bra burning frenzy it is vital that they should easily be able to buy bras that fit, are comfortable and are well made.

At present that is impossible and, in the remainder of this book, I will show why this is true and what can be done about it.

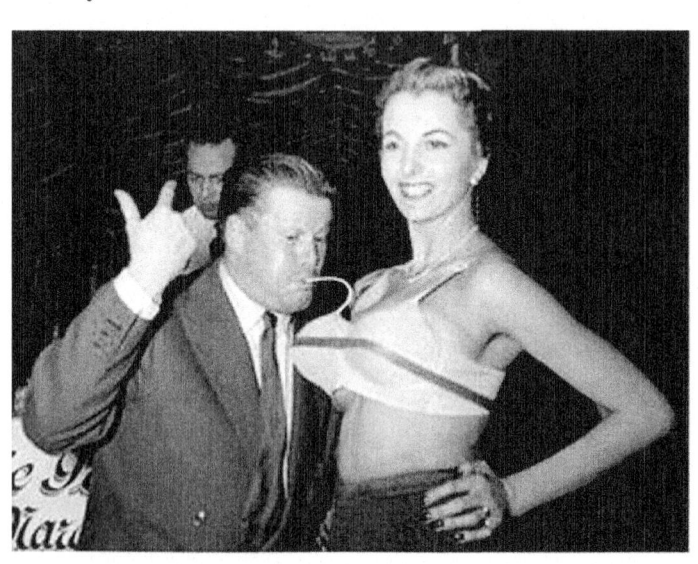

DID YOU KNOW THAT...

...the fashion for inflatable bras went into deflation when the introduction of high altitude intercontinental flights caused bra cups to explode?

3 A COMPARISON OF ONLINE BRA FITTING GUIDES

Introduction

The reason why so many bras fit very badly is because bra size advice is chaotic. There is no agreed standard that manufacturers and retailers work to so that simple measurements with a tape measure will ensure a comfortable, healthy and flattering fit.

There are video and pictures guides to obtaining a well fitting bra online. The best are the Figleaves [53] and Bravissimo websites [54]. These show how a bra should look and feel. The Figleaves website gives an excellent picture guide to choosing a bra using a simple questionnaire and the Bravissimo website has an excellent video.

Both websites advise buyers to '*...throw away the tape measure!*'

The problem of buying a good fitting bra has become even more difficult with bulk online bra suppliers.

For example, Amazon uses a bra fitting guide which is supposed to give an acceptable fit for the many makes of bra it supplies. However, the bra fitting guides on the manufacturers' websites often disagree considerably with the Amazon generic guide so it's impossible to get a consistent guide to bra size.

Before going further let's explain the concept of *'Sister Sizes'*. Two bra sizes are 'sister sizes' if their **Band** sizes differs by 2 inches and their **Cup** size is one different in the opposite direction. Thus, to go down a sister size reduce your **Band** size by two inches, but take your **Cup** size up one interval. You might go from a 36C to a 34D.

To go up a sister size increase your band size by 2 inches but go down one cup size. You might go from a 36C to a 38B. It is popularly claimed that women can wear comfortably bras which are 'sister' sizes.

It is certainly worth checking a 'sister' size when buying bras.

A systematic bra sizing system was introduced in the 1930s by Warners in the USA with four cup sizes called A, B, C and D.

However it was well into the 1950s before Britain followed this American practice.

British manufacturers were still using coy descriptions like 'junior' and 'medium' to describe breast fullness.

The Warner system was simple and produced bra size guidelines by using the following bust and frame information.

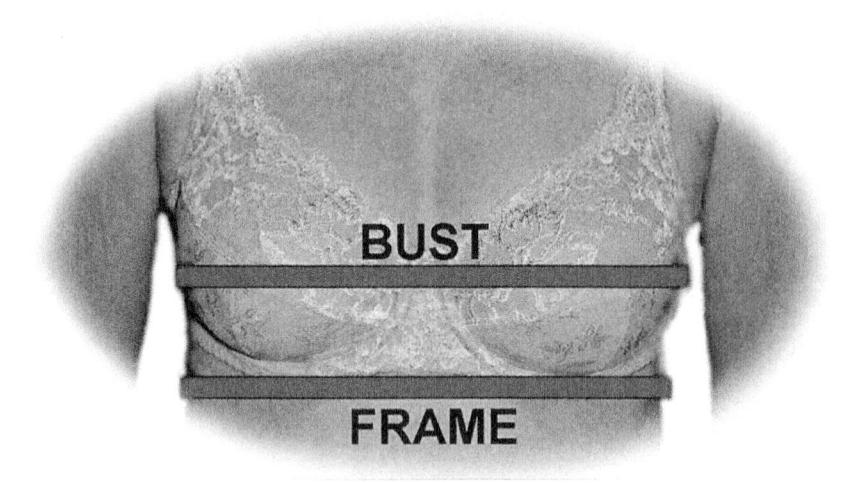

Referring to the picture above, the **'Frame'** measurement is made under the breasts whilst wearing a comfortable, well-fitting bra and the **'Bust'** measurement is made around the breasts at the largest position - usually over the nipples.

Making two measurements is usually all that is needed to come up with a bra size although one website recommends making three measurements, the third being above the breasts on the rib cage. This complication will be ignored here as it is very rarely used and

A COMPARISON OF ONLINE BRA-FITTING GUIDES

the 'Above Bust' measurement should be the same as the **'Frame'** measurement.

Most guides show the **'Bust'** measurements being made with the lady standing upright but at least one online guide recommends bending over so that the chest is parallel to the ground and the breasts are hanging down.

Confusion in terminology abounds. The summary below shows what the various measurements may be called.

BUST - Measurement around the largest part of the breasts whilst wearing a comfortable bra. Also called 'Over-Bust' on some websites

FRAME - The measurement around the ribcage immediately below the breasts. Also called 'Band', 'Under-Bust' or 'Back' on some websites

BAND - The numerical part of the bra size on the label. Also called 'Back' on some websites.

CUP - The letter identifying the cup size on the label.

GIRTH - The unstretched distance from hooks to eyes when a bra is laid out on the table. Also (wrongly) called the 'Band' on some websites.

In the rest of this book **Bust, Frame, Cup, Band** and **Girth** are written in bold and capitalised to show where they mean the measurement rather than just a general reference to a bra.

There is a widely propagated misconception that the **Band** is the circumference of the bra when slack. This is not the case and the slack circumference of a typical bra (the **Girth**) is between 6 and 10 inches less than the **Frame**.

In my comparisons of over twenty bra fitting online guides a small number of websites are American but ship to the UK. Unfortunately it is not always clear whether the bra sizes predicted are UK or US sizes.

The UK and US bra **Band** sizes are the same. However, the differences in the **Cup** size are slightly different.

Amazingly, even here websites disagree as to just what is the conversion between **Cup** sizes in the UK and US systems as shown below.

A COMPARISON OF ONLINE BRA-FITTING GUIDES

UK Cup Size	US Cup Size			
	Brasize.com [55]	85b [56]	Sizeguideuk [57]	Sizeguide [58]
AA			AA	
A	A/AA	AA	A	AA
B	B	A	B	A
C	C	B	C	B
D	D	C	D	C
DD	DD	D	DD/E	D
E	DDD/E	DD	DDD/F	DD
F	F	DDD/E	G	DDD/E
FF			H	
G	G	F	I	F
GG			J	

What a shambles!

I will now go through a summary of the online bra fitting guides briefly describing how they operate.

I will look at bra sizes up to **Cup** size GG. Anything larger requires a specialist fitting service. In addition, some online guides that have **Frame** sizes below about 28 inches have a different cup size rule and these sizes are not considered here. These are sometimes called 'teen' sizes which need special attention.

Sports bras also need specialist fitting although most women who buy a sports bra do so 'off the shelf'. The advice here may be used - with caution - for women who enjoy mild exercise.

Types of Online Bra Fitting Guides

There are broadly three systems in wide use for relating the measurements of **Bust** and **Frame** to bra size. These are used indiscriminatingly so that different retailers and websites come up with widely different predictions of your bra size.

The first of these bra sizing systems was the Warner Method [59].

A COMPARISON OF ONLINE BRA-FITTING GUIDES

When this method was introduced in the US in the 1930s the cup sizes were A, B, C and D. Today the average cup size is DD although the most popular size bra sold by Figleaves is currently 32F and so the old scale has been extended all the way up to N although online bra size guides usually stop before reaching that cup size.

The Warner scheme uses the following simple rules.

If the **Frame** measurement is even add 4 inches to get the **Band** size.

If the **Frame** measurement is odd add 5 inches to get the **Band** size.

The **Cup** size is related to the difference between the **Bust** and **Band** size as shown in the table below.

\multicolumn{11}{c	}{The 'Warner' Scheme}
FRAME	32	33	34	35	36	37	38	39	40	41	42
BAND	36	38	38	40	40	42	42	44	44	46	46
BUST minus BAND	<1	1	2	3	4	5	6	7	8	9	10
UK CUP	AA	A	B	C	D	DD	E	F	FF	G	GG
US CUP		AA	A	B	C	D	DD	E		F	

This obsolete system of bra sizing is still used by many retailers and online outlets.

Some retailers use their own unique systems. All use the **Bust** and **Frame** measurements as the basis for their predictions.

These alternatives to the 'Warner' system calculate the bra **Band** size from the **Frame** measurement by adding anything from zero to six inches.

We immediately see that the predicted bra **Band** sizes will cover a huge range - as indeed we will discover over the next few pages.

This not the end of your troubles.

A COMPARISON OF ONLINE BRA-FITTING GUIDES

The **Cup** size predictions are sometimes expressed in terms of the difference between the **Bust** and **Frame** measurements whilst other retailers use the difference between the **Bust** and **Band** to get the cup size.

Chaos!

What we are about to see is that putting the same **Bust** and **Frame** measurements into over twenty online bra fitting guides gives bra **Band** predictions differing by as much as FOUR inches and **Cup** sizes differing by an incredible FIVE cup sizes!

For example, putting a **Bust** measurement of 40 inches and a **Frame** measurement of 33 inches into over twenty online bra fitting guides gave predicted bra sizes ranging from a 'B' **Cup** right up to a 'G' **Cup**.

No wonder that 80% of you ladies are wearing badly fitting - and health threatening - bras!

The third 'system' for bra sizing is to throw away the tape measure and try on lots of bras - possibly under the eagle eye of a bra fitter - until a good well-fitting bra is found.

This system is used by Figleaves [84] and Bravissimo [87] and their website bra fitting guides are highly recommended.

Comparison of Online Bra Fitting Guides

The list below shows the online bra size prediction guides tested. The reference numbers in brackets guide you to the various websites listed at the end of this book.

Warner [59], La Senza [60], Amazon (UK) [61], Wikihow [62], Marks & Spencer [63], Avon [65], Ample Bosom [66], Beautiful Lingerie [67], Female First [68], Bare Necessities [69], 85b [70], Boobydoo [71], New Look [72], 007b [73], eBay [74], Silk Cocoon [75], Calculator.net [76], PSLingerie [77], Debenhams [78], mumsnet.com [79], Wisegeek.org [80], herroom.com [81], Ann Summers [82], House of Fraser [83], Figleaves [84], and Fashion World [85].

Five pairs of typical **Frame** and **Bust** measurements have been put into all the above online bra fitting guides and the predicted 'best' bra sizes have been compared.

Here are the **Frame** and **Bust** measurements put into the guides together with some of the bra sizes predicted by those guides.

A petite lady with small breasts -**Frame** 29 inches; **Bust** 31 inches. Predicted bra sizes range between 30AA and 34DD.

A medium sized lady with moderately full breasts -**Frame** 33 inches; **Bust** 40 inches. Predicted bra sizes range between 38B and 36G.

A medium sized lady with average breasts - **Frame** 34 inches; **Bust** 38 inches. Predicted bra sizes range between 38AA and 34D.

A larger lady with full breasts - **Frame** 38 inches; **Bust** 46 inches. Her predicted bra sizes range between 42D and 38H.

A larger frame lady with relatively small breasts - **Frame** 42 inches; **Bust** 46 inches. This lady's predicted bra sizes range between 46AA and 42D.

Clearly current online bra fitting guides using a tape measure as a guide are overwhelmingly useless and chaotic.

It is little wonder that 80% of women wear ill-fitting, uncomfortable and health-threatening bras!

Don't despair ladies because in chapter 5 I offer you a brand new bra sizing guide based on measurements of real women - not those skinny Photoshopped models you see in magazines. This new guide will usually get you within one bra **Band** size and one **Cup** size of your comfortable bra size.

I won't bore you with the detailed results of putting the five **Frame** and **Bust** combinations described above into twenty-one online bra sizing guides but I'll just tell you the best and worst.

In terms of predicting your **Band** size the most accurate were herroom.com [81], Wikihow [62], PSLingerie [77], Bare Necessities and mumsnet [79]. These averaged less than two inches error in recommended bra **Band** size.

The most inaccurate were the Debenhams [78], Ann Summers [82], Ample Bosom [66], Beautiful Lingerie [67] and Female First [68] all of which averaged over three inches error in **Band** size.

To be fair these results are not as bad as they might appear because the natural stretch in bra bands and the provision of two or more rows of hooks and eyes allows a degree of flexibility in choosing a bra band size.

All the twenty-one guides tested were within two bra **Bands**.

A COMPARISON OF ONLINE BRA-FITTING GUIDES

The real eye popping results were for the prediction of cup sizes. And when I say eye popping that what some of the recommended bras would do to you if you tried to wear them!

The best bra **Cup** size predictions were by Marks & Spencer [63], Amazon [61], Avon [65] and New Look [72]; all of who generally predicted **Cup** sizes to within about one size.

The losers were 85b [70], House of Fraser [83] and Female First [68], herroom.com [81] and calculator.net [76].

The worst of these guides averaged a massive three cup size error.

Incredible!

When looking at the best and worst overall bra fitting accuracy we find some surprising results.

For example, the herroom.com website sizing guide [81] performs best of the list on bra **Band** size but third from worst of **Cup** size.

So who are the overall winners and losers?

I have combined the results of testing the twenty-one websites against five body and breast sizes using a mathematical algorithm which I won't bore you with here.

Drumroll please!

Overall the least bad websites are Wikihow [62], herroom.com [81], Bare Necessities [69], mumsnet [79] and PSLingerie [77].

The websites who gave the least accurate recommendations overall for bra **Band** size and **Cup** size were 85b [70], House of Fraser [83], calculator.net [76] and Female First [68].

Summary

What a shambles online bra fitting guides are with you being offered bras differing by a huge five **Cup** sizes and four inches on bra **Band** size depending on which website you use.

The optimism of some websites is staggering.

For example, the Avon online bra sizing guide makes the following statement

'FACT: The majority of women out there are wearing the wrong bra size. Use this guide to help them find their perfect fit...'

In fact the Avon bra fitting guide uses the 'Obsolete' Warner system and covers a very limited range of bra sizes. My partner's very reasonable measurements of 34 inch **Frame** and 38 inch **Bust** are off the Avon scale.

What good is a bra fitting guide that does not cover the **Frame** and **Bust** measurements for 'real' women.

What is needed is a simple system using the **Frame** and **Bust** measurements to come up with a bra size which is the same for all online bra fitting guides.

This doesn't mean that a bra with that size will fit because, as we will see in the next two chapters, women with the same **Bust** and **Frame** measurements need different sized bras and bras with the same size printed on their labels can vary enormously in actual size and fit.

I will end this chapter with the excellent advice on the mumsnet website [79] which states

'To ensure you're buying a bra that fits properly, the best thing to do is head to an independent lingerie shop to be measured. In fact, Bravissimo (a store much-beloved by the larger-breasted of Mumsnet) long ago did away with the measuring tape and instead squints at your chest knowingly before handing over about 20 bras for you to try on until you find the perfect one.

DID YOU KNOW THAT...

...rubbing onions and garlic onto small breasts when a teenager is thought by some to make them grow larger?

My advice?

It won't work but you will never be dated by a vampire!

DID YOU KNOW THAT...

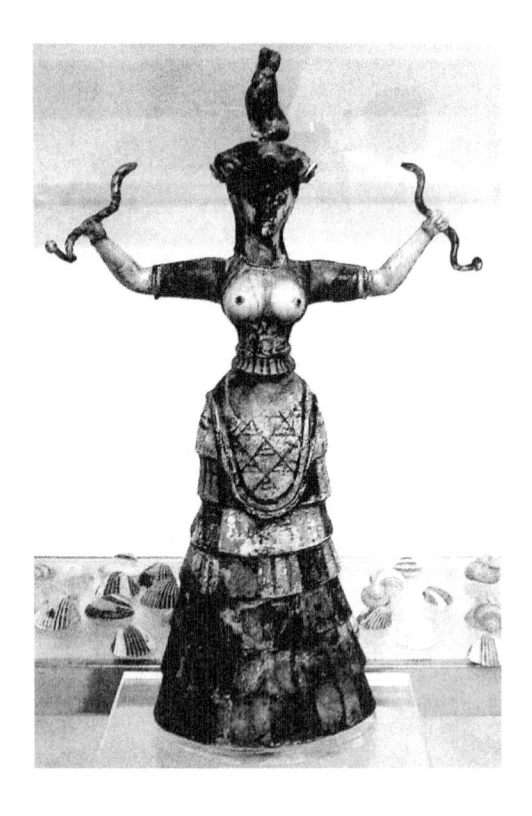

The Minoans (2,700 BCE - 1,500 BCE) were very 'breast orientated. The women wore 'bras' which pushed up their breasts so that they were fully exposed with a fine cleavage [99]

4. THE 'PORTSMOUTH' BRA STUDY

A major study of bra sizing reliability was published in 2012 by two researchers (Dr Jenny White and Dr Joanna Scurr) at Portsmouth University [86]. Dr White and Dr Scurr have very kindly given me access to their data and I have analysed the measurements in support of this book. I am greatly indebted to them for permitting me to use the data collected during their research.

They took 45 volunteers aged between 18 and 58 years with a wide range of breast sizes.

First the volunteers were asked what they considered their best bra size to be. Professional bra fitters then fitted the best selling Marks & Spencer non-padded, underwired T-shirt bra made from 78% Polyamide and 22% Elastane to each volunteer.

A comparison was made between the bra size the volunteers thought they were and their actual best bra size.

THE 'PORTSMOUTH' BRA STUDY

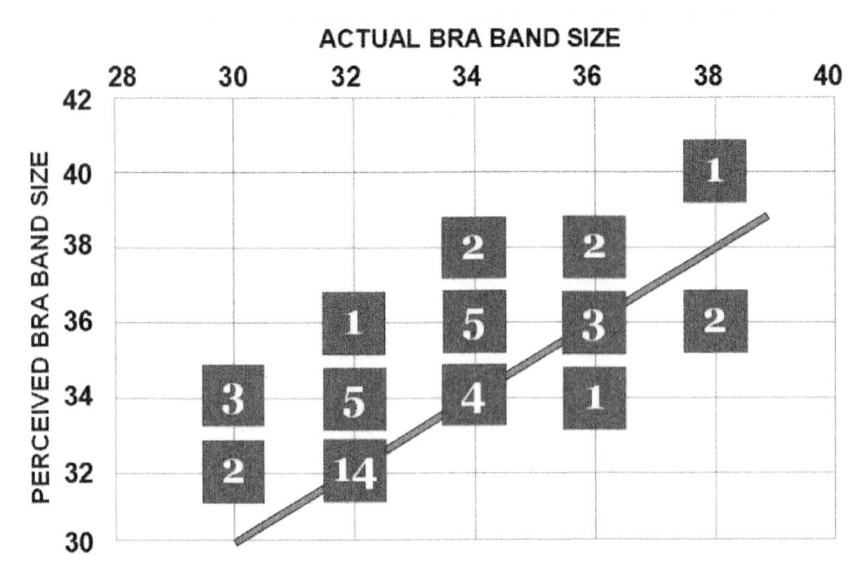

	ACTUAL BRA BAND SIZE						
PERCEIVED BRA BAND SIZE	28	30	32	34	36	38	40
42							
40						1	
38				2	2		
36			1	5	3		2
34		3	5	4	1		
32		2	14				
30							

The chart above shows a comparison of the volunteers' perceived bra band sizes with their actual band sizes as measured and fitted by professional bra fitters. The diagonal line shows where the perceived and correct bra bands agreed. The numbers on the chart show how many volunteers matched each measurement.

It can be seen that 47% of volunteers overestimated their band size, 47% perceived their bra band size correctly and the remaining 6% underestimated their bra band size. Some 13% of volunteers overestimated their bra band size by as much as four inches.

This means that many of these volunteers would be wearing bras which had loose bands. Because 80% of the weight of breasts is supported by the bra band gripping the ribcage, it follows that the straps on these lady's bras would be taking too much of the strain of supporting the breasts.

This in turn could be causing painful marks on the shoulders and consequential back and neck strain problems.

THE 'PORTSMOUTH' BRA STUDY

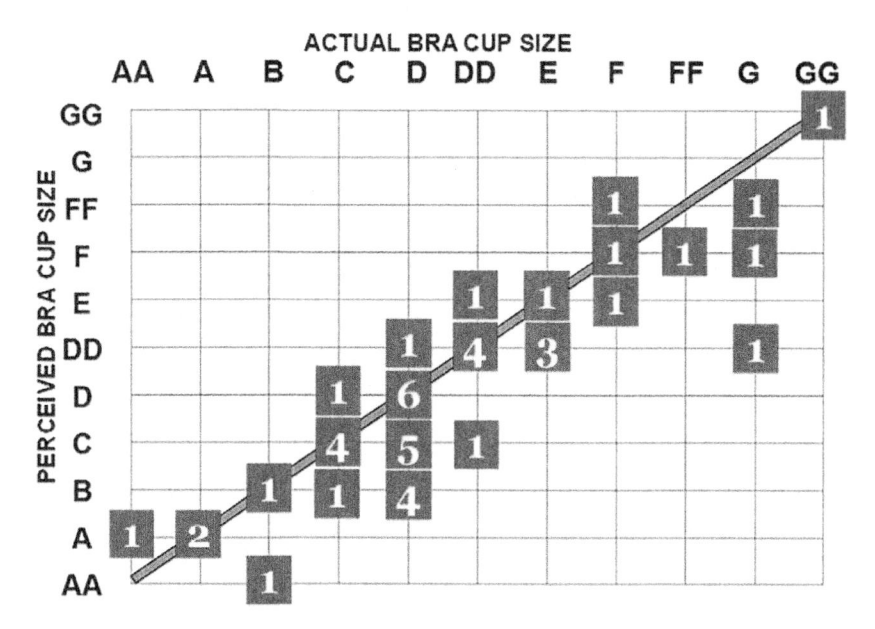

Above is a similar chart for the perceived and actual bra cup sizes.

In this case 44% of the volunteers underestimated their bra cup sizes, 44% had perceived bra cup sizes which were accurate and the remaining 12% overestimated their bra sizes.

One lady thought she was a DD cup but actually needed a G cup for comfort; an error of four cup sizes.

This means that many of these ladies were squeezing their breasts into cups which were much too small. Not only is this uncomfortable but the bra cup - and specifically the underwiring - will cut into the flesh and make breast health issues a possibility.

Overall, 71% of ladies in the study perceived their bra size wrongly.

In another analysis each volunteer's **Frame** and **Bust** measurements were recorded and then converted into **Band** and **Cup** measurements using a method which the researchers referred to as the 'Traditional Size' method.

As we have already seen, there are dozens of conflicting bra sizing guides of which the one used by Jenny White and Joanna Scurr is just one example. This conforms closely to the 1930s Warner method which is still widely used in online bra sizing guides.

THE 'PORTSMOUTH' BRA STUDY

The conversion used was:

If the **Frame** is even then add 4 inches otherwise add 5 inches. This is the **Band** size.

The **Cup** size was taken as 'A' for a **Bust** minus **Band** value of zero and one **Cup** size was added for each inch added reaching **Cup** size 'GG' for a nine inch difference between the **Bust** and **Frame** measurements.

It was found that the bra **Band** size predicted by the 'traditional' method could be up to six inches in error on the **Band** and the **Cup** as much as eight **Cup** sizes in error.

WOW!

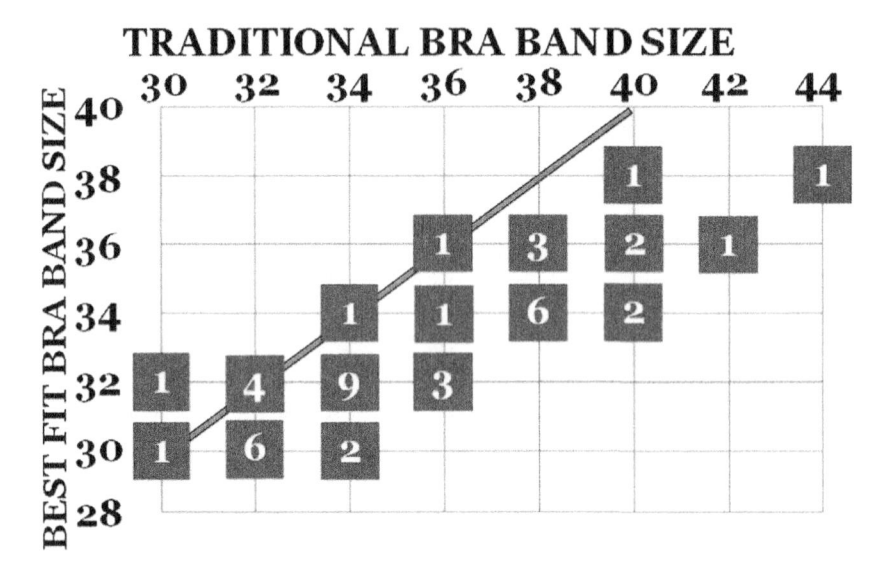

TRADITIONAL BRA BAND SIZE

BEST FIT BRA BAND SIZE	30	32	34	36	38	40	42	44
40								
38						1		1
36				1	3	2	1	
34			1	1	6	2		
32	1	4	9	3				
30	1	6	2					
28								

The above chart compares the bra **Band** size predicted by the 'Traditional' bra sizing procedure described above with the **Band** size found by the professional bra fitters.

The diagonal line shows where the Traditional **Band** Size would equal the Best Fit **Band** Size.

It can be seen that that only one volunteer had a **Band** size assigned by the professional bra fitter larger than her 'Traditional' bra **Band** size. The 'Traditional' Bra size predictions were overwhelmingly larger than the actual 'Best Fit' size particularly at larger sizes where the error was as large as six inches.

This means that ladies following the 'Traditional' bra sizing

('Warner') system would be trying on bras with a very loose band causing far too much breast weight on the straps with consequent back and neck pains as well as gouging marks on the shoulders.

We now turn to the prediction of **Cup** sizes by the 'Traditional' and the 'Best fit' methods.

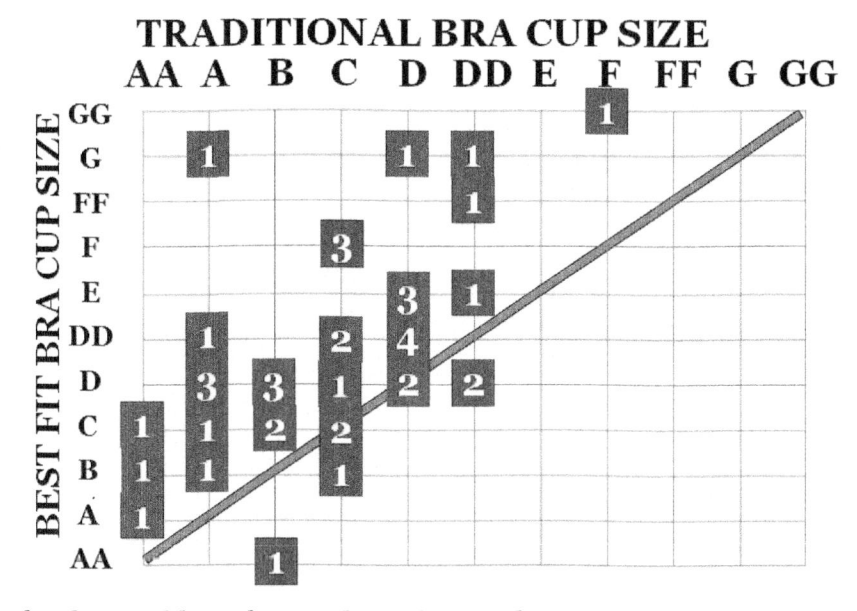

TRADITIONAL BRA CUP SIZE

(Chart: Traditional Bra Cup Size (AA A B C D DD E F FF G GG) vs Best Fit Bra Cup Size (AA A B C D DD E F FF G GG), with a diagonal line showing equality.)

The diagonal line shows where the 'Traditional' Bra Size would be equal to the 'Best Fit' cup size.

This chart is remarkable in showing the huge differences between the cup sizes predicted by the 'Traditional' Method and the actual 'Best Fit' cup size.

The 'Best Fit' cup sizes are overwhelmingly larger than the 'Traditional' Cup size with errors as large as eight cup sizes.

Notice that one lady's predicted bra **Cup** size using the 'Traditional' size guide was 'A' whereas she actually needed a 'G' cup!

Ladies using the 'Traditional' method of bra sizing would be squeezing their breasts into too small cups

No wonder that bra size guides perform so badly!

Not only do the online bra sizing charts disagree amongst themselves by huge margins, as seen in the previous chapter but we now see that concentrating on just one online bra sizing system

THE 'PORTSMOUTH' BRA STUDY

still gives massive discrepancies in prediction of the 'good bra' size.

In the next chapter I propose a new bra fitting scheme which, whilst it won't guarantee you the perfect fit (no guide ever can), will be much more reliable than any of the many guides studied so far.

5. A NEW BRA SIZING GUIDE

Bra sizing guides have to be simple.

Busy ladies do not want to make many measurements of their breasts and get involved in obscure mathematical calculations to come up with their correct bra size.

Two measurements (**Bust** and **Frame**) may not be sufficient to ensure a good fit but those two simple measurements ought to be enough to get close to the perfect bra fit. Then it's a case of trying different bra around the size I predict to find that perfect bra - if such an elusive object really does exist.

It's not rocket science to see from the previous charts that currently available bra sizing charts are useless with the exception of Bravissimo [87] and Figleaves [88]; neither of which rely on the tape measure to get a good fit.

My new bra sizing guide is simple to use and is based on the measurements and 'Best Fit' bras discovered by Dr Jenny White and Dr Joanna Scurr of Portsmouth University [89].

A NEW BRA SIZING GUIDE

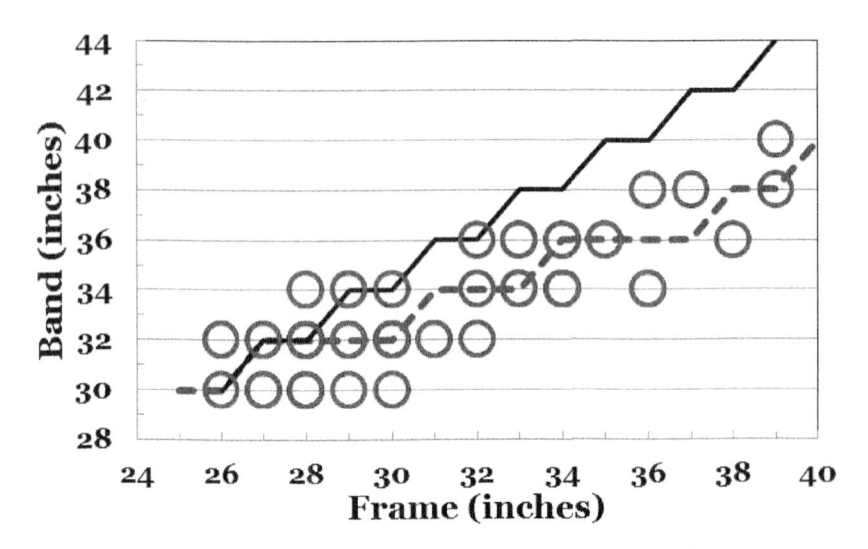

The above chart shows the 'Best Fit' **Band** values for bras found to be comfortable for women with the **Frame** sizes shown on the horizontal axis. (Remember that **Frame** size is the measurements under the breasts.)

Each circle represents the **Band** size found to be most comfortable for different **Frame** sizes. Remember - these results are for real women and represent reality; not some idealised, scrawny model in a Photoshopped advertisement.

The zigzagging upper line is the 'Traditional' relationship between **Frame** and **Band** sizes. That is to say band is **Frame** plus 4 inches if the **Frame** is an even number. Add 5 inches if the **Frame** is an odd number.

The zigzagging broken line is my proposal for a new relationship between **Frame** and **Band** size. This clearly represents the measurements on real ladies better than the 'Traditional' bra sizing system.

This can be summarised by the following table.

Frame	26	27	28	29	30	31	32	33
Band	30	32	32	32	32	34	34	34
Frame	34	35	36	37	38	39	40	41
Band	36	36	36	36	38	38	40	40

A NEW BRA SIZING GUIDE

Now for a new **Cup** size scheme.

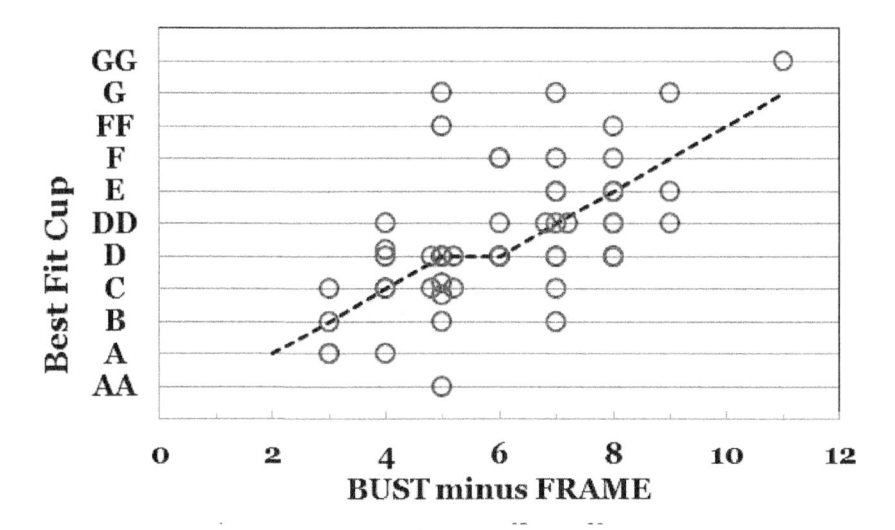

This shows the 'Best Fit' **Cup** size plotted against the **Bust** minus **Frame** measurement for the 'Portsmouth Study' database.

The new relationship between **Cup** size and the difference between **Bust** and **Frame** sizes is shown by the dotted line on the chart above. This is represented by the values in the table below.

BUST minus FRAME	2	3	4	5	6	7	8	9	10	11
UK CUP	A	B	C	D	D	DD	E	F	FF	G
US CUP	AA	A	B	C	C	D	DD	E	E	F

Now for the acid test of this new scheme - how does it compare with other bra sizing schemes?

The data collected during the 'Portsmouth Study' [91] produced 'Best Fit' bra sizes for combinations of **Frame** and **Bust** sizes for 45 volunteers. A selection of these **Frame** and **Bust** sizes have been input into a random selection of online bra sizing guides to obtain predicted bra sizes.

In addition, the new scheme recommended above was used to predict the Best Fit bra sizes found by the Portsmouth researchers.

A NEW BRA SIZING GUIDE

On the following charts the circles are my new bra sizing scheme predictions for the given **Frame** and **Bust** measurements. The squares are the predictions for typical online bra sizing schemes and the triangles are typical results for real ladies.

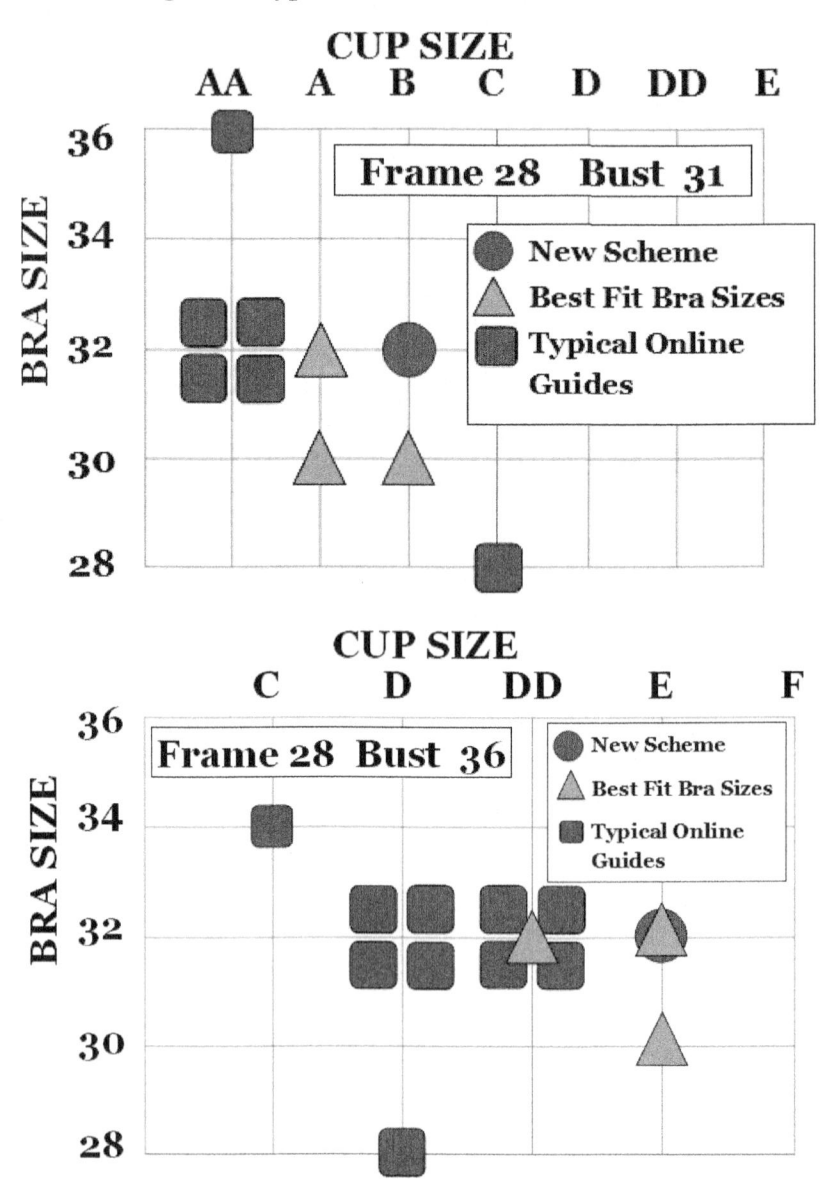

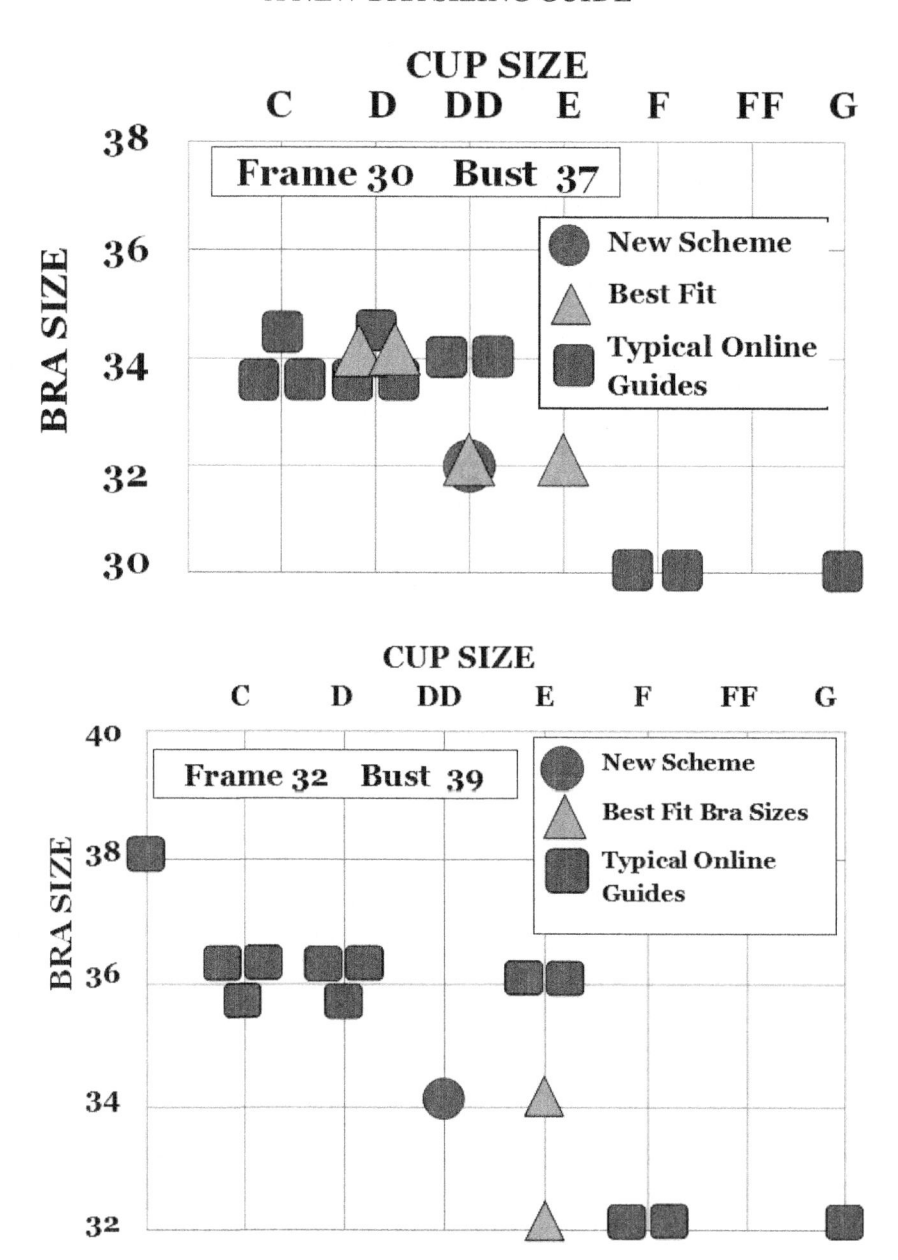

A NEW BRA SIZING GUIDE

A NEW BRA SIZING GUIDE

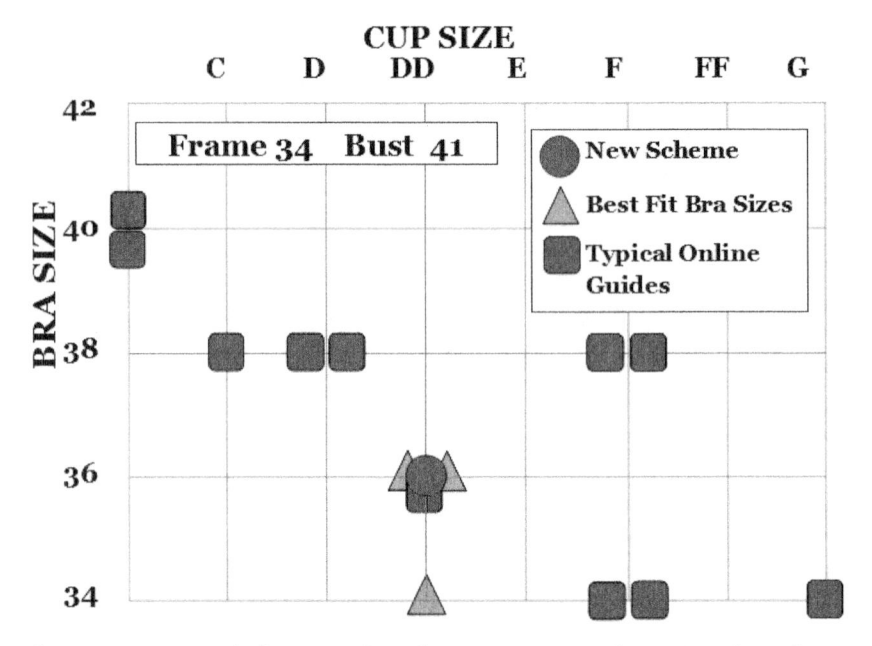

CUP SIZE: C, D, DD, E, F, FF, G
BRA SIZE: 34, 36, 38, 40, 42

Frame 34 Bust 41

Legend:
- ● New Scheme
- ▲ Best Fit Bra Sizes
- ■ Typical Online Guides

The proximity of the circular data points to the triangles shows clearly that the new bra sizing scheme much more accurately represents the bra sizes of real ladies than the online guides as shown by the square symbols.

On all the above five charts the new scheme predicts within one **Band** size and one **Cup** size the best fit bra sizes found by the University of Portsmouth researchers.

By comparison, the online bra fitting guides can be as much as four **Band** sizes and four **Cup** sizes in error.

Having found hopelessly unreliable bra sizing information online you will now want to buy a bra.

Your problems are not at an end because bras with the same size on the label will be found to vary enormously in their **Band** and **Cup** sizes.

6. HOW DOES A BRA WORK?

Bras are complicated devices which have to combine comfort, practicality, cheapness, support, flexibility, appearance and durability. Unfortunately, the aggressively profit-driven bra industry is, with a few significant exceptions, only really interested in cheapness and appearance. Why else would some manufactures make bras with sexy - but scratchy - lacy cups but not line them?

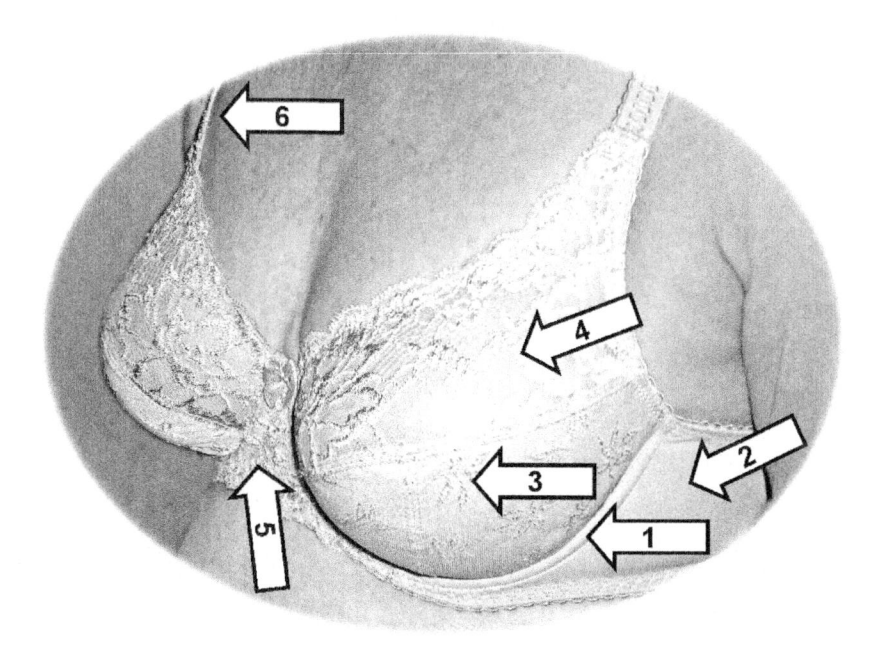

The picture shows the main parts of a bra. In some bras there are fewer parts - such as a T-shirt bra where the cup is a single

HOW DOES A BRA WORK?

moulded cup. In other bras, such as those with large cup sizes, there may be extra parts to the cups to provide more support and transmit the weight of the breasts less painfully to the band.

The parts shown on the picture above are as follows.

1. The underwiring.

Some bras have no underwiring but these usually have a stiff narrow stitched band under the cups which achieves the same purpose. The underwiring should fit snugly on the boundary between the ribcage and the breast tissue without resting on the breast tissue. If the underwire is too small the breast tissue will be trapped which is not only painful but it can cause health problems - possibly serious.

About 80% to 90% of the weight of a breast is carried through the cup material to the underwiring. The underwiring is the intermediate structure that transmits the breast weight to the band.

The picture below proves what I have just written. I fixed an underwired 36DD bra cup to a vertical wooden board and placed a water-filled balloon in the cup weighing 1 kg which is the weight of a 36DD breast.

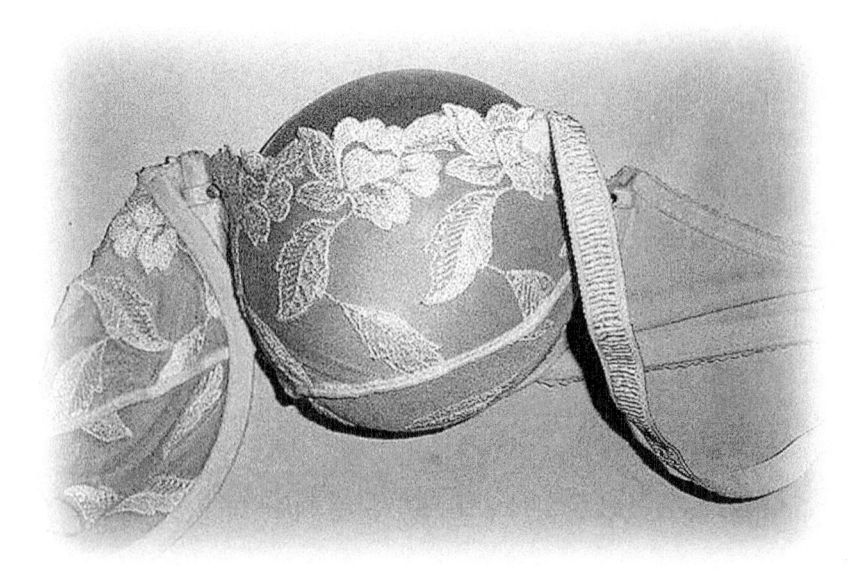

It can be seen that the cup is supporting the weight of the water-filled balloon with the bra strap slack. All of the 1 kg weight is

HOW DOES A BRA WORK?

perfectly supported by the underwire.

An odd feature of the underwiring is that it is flat.

Lay a bra on a flat surface and hold the wire down gently. It has to lay snug on the ribcage without cutting into the flesh or sticking out away from the flesh because this transfers extra force elsewhere on the ribcage.

So, is your ribcage flat?

Of course not!

Take your oldest bra and remove the wire. Now try to fit it in the fold of a breast where the breast tissue meets the ribcage. This is called the Inframammary Fold. The chances are it doesn't sit snugly in the fold and has to be pressed down against the ribcage.

So, why are bras not made with underwires that are shaped in three dimensions to fit snugly without creating a painful pinch point?

Could it be that a bra wire curved in three dimensions is a few pence or cents more expensive to manufacture?

Flat underwires enable the bra to be packed flat which is easier to distribute and stack on shop displays.

Surely manufacturers would not be so unfeeling and profit-driven that would put comfort and health of the bra wearers before relatively trivial extra cost?

Of course they would!

2. The band

This strip of elasticated fabric carries over 80% of the weight of the breasts. The weight of each breast is carried by the cup to the underwiring and thence to the band supporting the underwiring.

In order to carry the weight of the breasts the band has to grip the ribcage. The heavier the breasts the more the band has to dig into the flesh of the ribcage to stop the bra sliding down. For this reason the areas of bra bands need to be increased as the weight of the breasts increase.

The band is often fitted with a sticky strip of the type used to hold up suspender-less 'holdup' stockings.

HOW DOES A BRA WORK?

3. The Lower Part of the Cup

The lower part of the cup carries the weight of the breast and transmits this to the under-wiring - see the photograph above.

This cup is usually spherical in shape. This is because a sphere exerts the same pressure everywhere like a balloon. Were the cup material deformed into a substantially different shape from a sphere then the pressure on the breasts would vary from point to point causing discomfort, stress and a very strange appearance!

4. The Upper Part of the Cup

This does very little. Only 10% - 20% of the weight of each breast is carried via the material above the nipple to the strap.

The fact that bra straps can be slipped over your shoulders and the upper part of the cup material be rolled down without much change to the breast shape shows that the upper part of the cup is almost redundant.

Hence we can buy demi-cup, strapless underwired bras - at least in sizes DD or less - without the upper cup area being present.

5. The Bridge or Gore

This connects the cups together. The shape of the Bridge/Gore determines the force on the under-wire and, if this small part of the bra is incorrectly designed, the under-wire will be distorted causing pain and stress. For a well-designed bra the Bridge/Gore should lie flat on the rib cage without digging in and without gaping.

6. The Straps

The straps support little of the weight of the breasts; less than 20% and usually about 10%. This means that the straps play a very small part in the working of the bra. This in turn means that bra straps that cut into the shoulder flesh are much too tight.

7. BRA BUYING PROBLEMS

Now that you are convinced that current online bra fitting guides are generally useless, it's time to ignore them and buy a new bra without their woefully bad advice.

One technique is to put on your current best bra and use the Figleaves [92] or Bravissimo [93] online fitting guides to point you towards buying a new bra that fits.

An alternative is to go out and buy a bra the same as the one you are wearing. This is particularly favoured by bigger breasted ladies because finding a good fit is more difficult and Bravissimo, for example, has a reputation for reliable large bra sizing.

Yet another option is to use my new bra fitting guide from chapter 5 to get you into the right ballpark to start trying on bras.

So, armed with your 'perfect fit' bra size in your diary you set off to the shops or start buying online.

What you will find is that some bras with your 'Best Fit' size on the label fit moderately well whilst others may be close but not close enough and some will be uselessly large or small.

Why is this?

Well, Carol Ann Dunbar who is an underwear model found out.

She was sent by Daily Mail reporter Marianne Power to expert bra fitter Dita Summerfield from Rigby & Peller, underwear fitters to the Queen [94].

Dita found that Carol's best fitting bra size was a 32C. Carol had

BRA BUYING PROBLEMS

believed she was a small 'B' cup.

Carol started with an H&M Multi-function push up bra. The 32C was too tight, 34C fit but hurt. Carol stated

'What a disaster! These were the most uncomfortable bras I've ever tried on. The 32C was so narrow I could hardly do it up, and the underwiring was so harsh it dug in and made my skin red. The 34C fitted but was still uncomfortable.'

Carol then tried on a Next plunge bra and found the 32C was far too small such that she could not fasten the bra at the back.

A size 32D was better but far from perfect. Dita Summerfield considered that a 30D would have been better but Next did not stock bras smaller than size 32.

A BHS Secrets range bra at size 32C was hopeless but a 32D was a reasonable fit.

A Marks & Spencer 32C bra suffered from tight wiring but a 30D fit perfectly.

The John Lewis 32C bra was too wide but a 30D fitted perfectly.

A Debenhams 32C bra was a really comfortable bra and it fitted perfectly. However, the comment was made that the staff were very rude.

'Nobody offered to help us and the shop assistant was quite brusque with us, getting annoyed that we wanted to use the same changing room.'

This small survey of high street bras showed that Carol thought she was a size 32B but was professionally fitted out as a 32C.

The bras that fitted her best in her search were 30D, 32C and 32D.

Some 32C bras were *'way too small', 'hopeless', 'too tight', 'too wide'* or *'perfect'* showing how bras vary considerably even though they have the same size on the label.

What women need is a single consistent bra sizing guide that is used by all online and in-store bra fitting services. Bras must then be made that fit those sizes.

It's not rocket science and yet it has not been done.

Wikipedia cites [95] a shift in styling and advertising to the detriment of women's comfort and health as follows-

BRA BUYING PROBLEMS

'*Manufacturers' marketing and advertising often appeals to fashion and image over fit, comfort and function. Since about 1994, manufacturers have re-focused their advertising, moving from advertising functional brassieres that emphasize support and foundation, to selling lingerie that emphasize fashion while sacrificing basic fit and function, like linings under scratchy lace.*'

In addition, manufacturers create 'vanity sizes' and deliberately put the wrong labels in their bras.

Branding the system 'a scam', New York boutique owner Linda Becker [96] has said that modern bras are labelled with smaller back sizes and larger cup sizes so that the wearer thinks she is not only slimmer around the rib cage but more buxom around the breasts.

She says women who have not been fitted in some time could easily be wearing a poorly-fitting bra, as many manufacturers have changed the sizing without warning customers.

In an interview with ABC News, Ms Becker, who calls herself 'The Bra Lady', said:

'*I realized all the companies about 10 years ago changed all the sizes without telling us. They 'vanity sized' it, they wanted you to think your back was smaller and your breasts were bigger.*'

Describing the scale of the problem, she says that what was once labelled a 36D is now often labelled a 32G.

She said that in order to ensure a good fit, every woman should be fitted by a professional, and replace their bras every six months.

Until bra manufacturers and retailers get together and adopt a consistent guide scheme (such as mine) and make bras to the same sizing templates the overwhelming majority of women will continue to suffer in badly fitting, pinching, bulging and health threatening bars.

And yet, many women still buy bras to give themselves abnormal breast shapes and cleavages in the delusion that this is more important than having an attractive personality.

In March 2012 the UK's Channel 4 transmitted a TV documentary which included a visit to a Chinese 'Bra Town' where identical bras were being manufactured for various UK stores where they were sold for widely different prices; the price depending on the name on the label [97].

BRA BUYING PROBLEMS

So, you are in a shop fitting room with a pile of potential bras which may be different sizes but with the same 'size' printed on the label. The only option is to try them on and home in on the bra that fits best.

Use the next two pictures to check your bra fit which follow the best of the online bra fitting guide recommendations (Figleaves and Bravissimo).

There are eight checkpoints to satisfy.

It doesn't take a degree in advanced mathematics to realise that the chance of finding a bra that satisfies all eight key features at the same time - and looks attractive - is very small.

Either some compromise will be necessary or you will spend a long time trying on bras at several retailers. Clearly this is where buying online is a problem because you may not feel like ordering twenty bras and sending nineteen back.

This is also a problem when using a bra fitting service because the fitter may push you (literally!) into a bra that is not suitable because there is nothing in stock that fits correctly

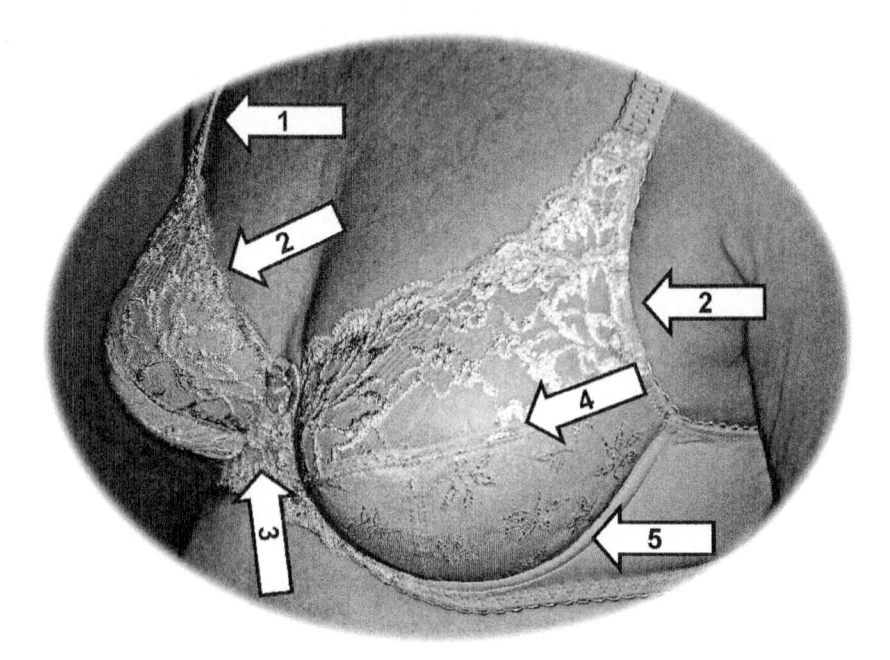

Check 1 The straps should not dig in or even feel as though they are exerting more than a comfortable amount of pressure.

BRA BUYING PROBLEMS

Remember that bra straps support no more than 20% of the weight of your breasts. If the straps feel at all uncomfortable loosen them or try a bra with wider straps.

Check 2 The lines where the bra cups meet the flesh should be smooth with no gaping or pressure on the skin. The upper part of the bra cup plays only a small role in supporting your breasts so there should be no uncomfortable pressure. The line from the bra cup to the ribcage should be smooth - no bulging and no gaps showing through your top. The line of the edge of your bra cups should be invisible under a smooth thin top.

Check 3 The central Bridge or Gore should lay comfortably flat on your ribcage with no digging in or gaping.

Check 4 The bra cups should be smooth and rounded like part of a ball. A mathematician will tell you that a bra cup with a uniform curvature is the most comfortable. Avoid cups that push and squeeze your breasts into unnatural shapes.

Certainly avoid bra cups with a thick seam running across the middle. It is very much of a 'turn off' because a seam line sticking out on your otherwise smooth dress or sweater profile is not attractive. However, when buying a bra with smooth seam-free cups you may have to go up a cup size [98].

Check 5 The underwire should lie comfortably in the Infra-mammary Fold which is where the breast tissue meets the ribcage skin. Get this wrong and you will be squeezing the wire hard and trapping breast tissue. If the wire sits too low it will not be supporting the breast correctly. Remember - 80% of the weight of each breast is held by the underwire. It is very important to get this right.

BRA BUYING PROBLEMS

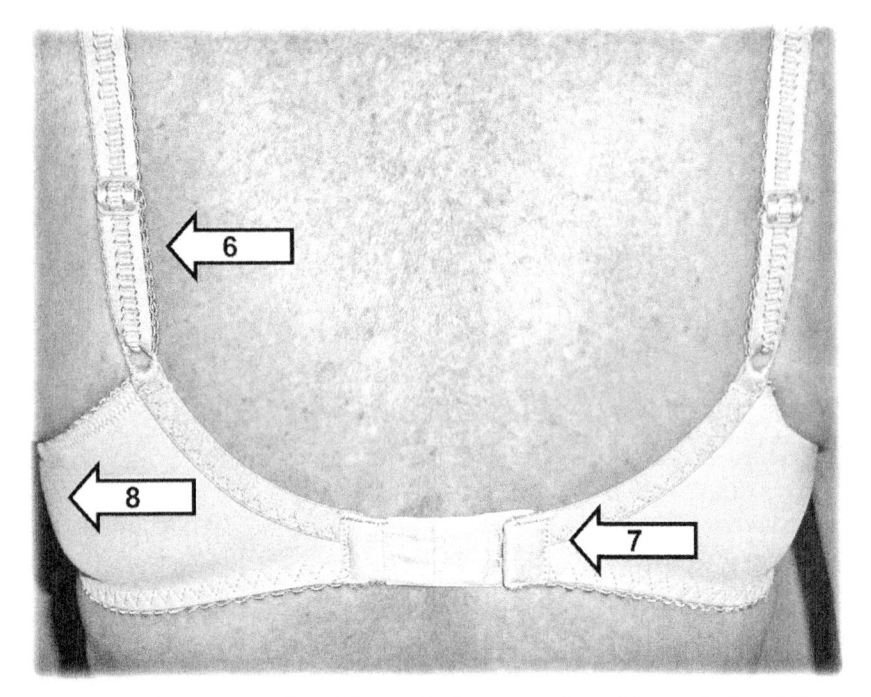

Check 6 The straps should not feel uncomfortable and should run straight up and down your back unless you are wearing a bra that has an integrated back or a cross strap back. These are usually sports bras.

Check 7 The back of the band should lie horizontal about 4 inches below the line of the armpits. If the bra band curves up or down over your back the bra is either the wrong band size or the straps are pulled too tight.

Reach around and pull the band away from your spine with a thumb. The band should be pulled 2 inches if the bra band is correctly fitting. Slacker than this and the straps will be carrying too much breast weight. Tighter and your bra will be painful and a health risk.

The clasps should be on the loosest setting to allow for the bra going saggy with age.

Check 8 The bra band should not exert uncomfortable pressure on the underarm ribcage and the edges of the band should never leave red marks. This is where some of the lymph drains toxins from the breast and this pressure must be kept as low as possible. There should be no bulging at the edges of the bra band.

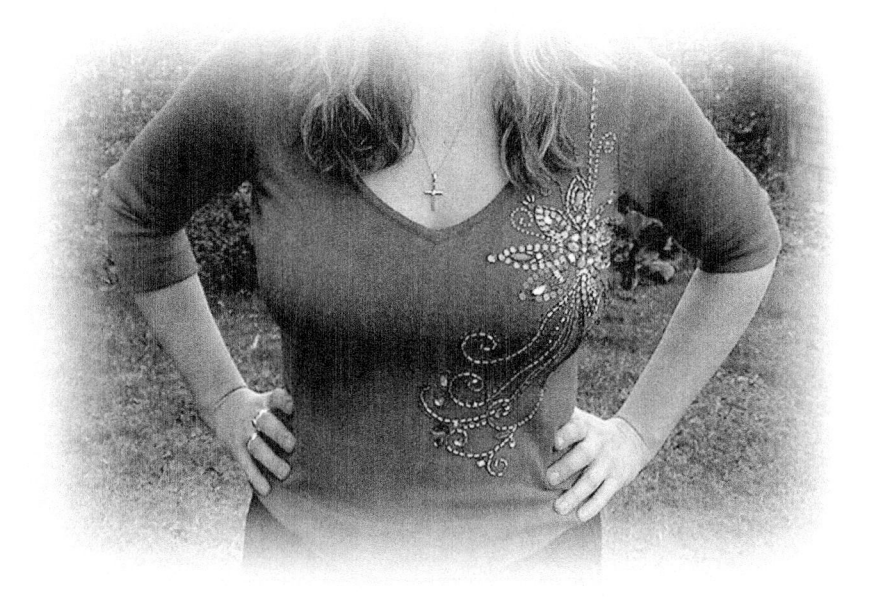

Your bra should be invisible under an opaque top as seen above. No lines or ridges showing where the bra cups end, no strap marks, a smooth transition across the Bridge/Gore between the cups, no ugly bulging out of the bra band under the armpits and no sign of the bra back band.

If this is what you see in a mirror then your bra probably is a good comfortable fit.

DID YOU KNOW THAT...

...bra manufacturers manufacture bras with so-called invisible straps for wearing with off-the-shoulder dresses. However, they often use shiny plastic which glares as it reflects light. If they used a transparent but non-reflective material the straps would truly be invisible.

BRA BUYING PROBLEMS

DID YOU KNOW THAT...

...during World War I women were stopped from buying corsets? This freed up so much steel that in one year 28,000 tons were saved enabling two warships to be built.

DID YOU KNOW THAT...

...the front fastening bra has almost disappeared from the shops? 'Front loaders' are much easier for their wearers to do up but more difficult for their lovers to undo.

Why have they largely vanished from the shops?

8. PULLING IT ALL TOGETHER

In this chapter we review what we have learned, what we have unlearned, what we never knew and are happy not to have known.

First of all there is no evidence that wearing a bra is beneficial to health. It is not a garment performing a task that compliments natural bodily health.

It is a binding garment although a less extreme form of body binding than the Chinese did to women's feet a century ago where the 'ideal' foot was a mere three inches in length. However, binding women's breasts is just as illogical.

Breasts have, over the centuries, been pushed up, flattened, squeezed together and strapped into a garment which is known to cause breast pain and may cause cysts and possibly even breast cancer by cutting off the natural flow of lymphatic fluids around the breasts.

Bra wearing has no medical benefits.

The reason many women refuse to cast off their bras is because they fear their breasts will sag.

They won't.

In fact bra wearing encourages sagging and leaving off a bra makes breasts firmer and perkier.

Carefully controlled medical studies have shown that women with breast pain and cysts enjoyed a 50% reduction in days with 'moderate' and 'severe' breast pain after they left off their bras.

PULLING IT ALL TOGETHER

Overall, for all women in the test there was a reduction of 7% in days with pain.

The survey of about 5,000 women by Sydney Ross Singer and Soma Grismaijer shown a very strong correlation between the average number of hours each day spent wearing a bra and the incidence of breast cancer.

The experimenters argued that bras cause breast cancer and this is because the tightness of bras restricts the flow of lymphatic fluids in the breast resulting in the build up of toxins.

Medical professionals who argue against the survey results and the mechanism of toxin build up broadly dismiss the survey by arguing that the results were not published in a peer reviewed science journal.

However, scientific research is not diminished in stature and validity because it has not been approved by a cartel of the scientific elite. It typically costs over $2,500 to get a research paper published in a quality journal [100].

As one anonymous professor has stated

'The review process is a playground of promoting personal opinions, rather than evaluating the actual science' [101]

Also, scientists can be terribly wrong for a very long time as has been demonstrated by the scandal of the treatment of gastric ulcers.

The most damning 'evidence' against the perceived link between bra wearing and breast cancer was the claim that women who had their breast lymph nodes removed were no more susceptible to developing breast cancer than those who didn't.

But then Singer and Grismaijer alleged that this 'evidence' was not published in a peer reviewed science journal.

A common argument against the hypothesis of Singer and Grismaijer is that

'...*there is no evidence that bras cause breast cancer*'.

Absence of evidence is not evidence of absence.

If Singer and Grismaijer are the only people to have carried out a survey to look for a link then the absence of evidence against their results is simply attributable to the fact that nobody has looked for that link not that the link has been sought by other researchers and has not been found.

However, there are reports in science journals in Chinese, Spanish and French that show a danger of developing cancer as a result of bra wearing.

It is claimed by cancer researchers and experts that breast cancer correlates with several well-established factors such as number of pregnancies, smoking, weight (Body Mass Index), genetic susceptibility, exposure to toxins, etc.

Could it not be that overweight women wear their bras longer each day than slim women and this is the reason why there is an apparent relationship between bra wearing and breast cancer?

Unfortunately, nobody appears to have looked for a relationship between breast cancer susceptibility, body weight and bra wearing habits. Had this been done we would not still be arguing, eighteen years after Singer and Grismaijer published their survey results, about whether bra wearing really is a contributor to breast cancer.

What cannot be denied is that the Singer and Grismaijer survey shows a very clear - even spectacular - relationship between bra wearing habits and breast cancer incidence.

Traditionally living Fijian women don't wear bras and do not suffer breast cancer. Those who become westernised and wear bras as part of their adopted life style suffered breast cancer rates similar to Caucasian females.

With around 450,000 women suffering each year from breast cancer why have the definitive studies not been performed to answer this essential question -

'Does wearing a bra increase the risk of breast cancer?'

The multi-million dollar bra industry will not allow a campaign to succeed that casts doubt on the safety of their products. It fights back by claiming that unless girls are measured for, and fitted with, bras starting around the age of nine and extending all the rest of their life, then there will be terrible penalties to be paid of which sagging is one.

This scare tactic combined with the ruthless marketing of bras as sex garments means that very few women are going to enjoy the pleasures and health benefits of going bra-less.

PULLING IT ALL TOGETHER

So, despite all you have read you still want to stick with your bra?

Many of the online and department store bra fitting guides have been shown here to be unacceptably inaccurate except for Figleaves and Bravissimo. Putting your measurements into a typical guide will suggest bras up to four inches too big or too small on the bra band size and up to four cup sizes in error.

I have invented a new bra sizing guide developed with generous assistance from researchers at the UK University of Portsmouth. This is more accurate than any existing bra fitting guide and will put you into the right ballpark to choose a bra.

However, the next pitfall is that bras carrying the same sizes on the labels can be widely different in actual size. This is 'vanity sizing' where manufacturers deliberately misrepresent their bras to make the wearer believe they are slimmer and sexy than they really all.

If manufacturers use my new bra sizing guide and manufactured bras to the same agreed template then badly fitting bras would be much rarer.

By following my health advice (chapter 2), using my new bra sizing guide (chapter 5) and persuading manufacturers to stop 'vanity sizing' and making bras to consistent shapes and sizes (chapter 7), millions of women, who choose not to give up bra wearing, could have comfortable bras, better health and a greatly improved lifestyle.

They could better pick up, carry their children and cuddle them without breast pains.

Isn't that worth it?

Spread the word ladies!

9 ABOUT THE AUTHOR

I have a degree in Physics from London University and another degree in Environmental Science from the Open University. My career has mainly been in Oceanography and Underwater Acoustics. Clearly, I am not qualified to write about breasts as a result of my career and academic studies.

However, I can claim over sixty years of enthusiastic interest in breasts and bras excluding those infant years when my interest was more nutritional than sexual.

I do not wear bras so I can accept no responsibility for the consequences - good or bad - from taking the advice on buying and wearing a bra given in this publication

My experience has not always been recognized as shown by my letter below published in the Dorset Evening Echo on Christmas Eve 1989.

Letter to the Dorset Echo

When experience just ain't enough

I note with outrage the advertisement for a manageress at the Weymouth Contessa shop. This is blatant discrimination since we men are not allowed to apply!

Men have far more experience of getting ladies out of and into their underwear than any women.

Indeed, I can claim over 40 years' experience of struggling to help females of all shapes and sizes out of and back into bra cups sizes ranging from A to FF - as

ABOUT THE AUTHOR

well as coping with lower garments ranging from thongs to fully-elasticated thermal drawers.

It is blatant sex discrimination to ban me and other men like me, with our vast experiences, from this job at Contessa. And, had I been allowed to apply for this job, I would gladly have done it fulltime for no pay.

G. Kirby

Weymouth

Dorset

10 FURTHER READING

Thomas, Pauline Weston *'History of Bras and Girdles'* http://tinyurl.com/pmoxcyo Retrieved 01 January 2014

Power, Marianne, Daily Mail online *'So that's why your bras never fit!'* http://tinyurl.com/798vyyp Retrieved 5 January 2014

Seigel, Jessica *'Bent Out Of Shape - Why is it so hard to find the perfect bra?'* http://www.jessicaseigel.com/articles/bra.shtml Retrieved 13 January 2014

Uhlig, Robert *'Engineers famous for their wobble help build £2m bra'* http://tinyurl.com/nz2rwv7 Retrieved 13 January 2014

Anon, *'Bras I Hate And Love'* http://tinyurl.com/nt2dwzn Retrieved 13 January 2014 A blog by a 30HH lady who blogs about bigger bras with wit and wisdom.

Becky's Boudoir *'Bra Fit Problems - Bust Shape and Wires'* http://tinyurl.com/ouvccvw Retrieved 7 February 2014

Herroom - 'Anatomy *of a bra - How bras are made to fit your unique shape'* http://tinyurl.com/pf2gqz6 Retrieved 13 January 2014

Wikipedia - Brassiere - https://en.wikipedia.org/wiki/Brassiere Retrieved 13 January 2014

Wikipedia - Measuring Bras - https://en.wikipedia.org/wiki/Brassiere_measurement Retrieved 13 January 2014

FURTHER READING

Advice from Susan Nethero, - see. http://tinyurl.com/ozat7pb

Singer, Sydney Ross and Grismaijer, Soma, *'Dressed To Kill: The Link Between Breast Cancer and Bras'* Avery Publishing Corp. New York 1995 ISBN 0-89529-664-0

Singer, Sydney Ross and Grismaijer, Soma Bra and Cancer blog http://www.killerculture.com/breast-cancer-is-preventable/

Claiborne Ray, *'Bras and Cancer'* A Criticism of the Singer and Grismaijer study. http://tinyurl.com/o98ujf3

Pederson, Stephanie *'Bra: A Thousand Years of Style, Support and Seduction'* (Available from Amazon)

Dominy, Katie *'Contemporary Lingerie Design'* (Available from Amazon)

Hawthorne, Rosemary *'Bras: A Private View'* (Available from Amazon)

The 'Bra Free' website which has lots of encouraging facts to support women who choose to go bra free http://www.brafree.org/faq.html Retrieved 12 January 2014

'Bras Mess With Your Sleep and Immune System' http://tinyurl.com/bqapk6y Retrieved 21 January 2014

'Is your bra making you ill?' Guardian Online 2 December 2008 http://tinyurl.com/3svpjef Retrieved 12 January 2014

'Are you wearing the right bra? We go back to boob school' UK Daily Mirror online 26 April 2013 http://tinyurl.com/pmtw5vc Retrieved 12 January 2014

'Prevention and Treatment of Fibrocystic Breast Disease' Ralph L. Reed, Ph.D http://all-natural.com/fibrocys.html Retrieved 12 January 2014 This includes a large amount of anecdotal evidence relating bra wearing and breast health problems.

Cheree Berry 'Hoorah *for the Bra: A Perky Peek at the History of the Brassiere'* Available from Amazon

Susan Nethero *'Bra Talk' - Myths and Facts'* Kindle eBook.

Florence Williams *'Breasts: Natural and Unnatural History'*. Kindle eBook.

Sanders-Steel, Debra *'The Ultimate Bra Fitting Guide'* Outskirts Press Inc. (2013) Available from Amazon

11. REFERENCES

1. Singer, Sydney Ross and Grismaijer, Soma *'Dressed To Kill: The Link Between Breast Cancer and Bras'* Avery Publishing Corp. New York 1995 ISBN 0-89529-664-0

2. Thomas, Pauline Weston *'History of Bras and Girdles'* http://tinyurl.com/pmoxcyo Retrieved 01 January 2014

3. Wikipedia copyright-free image. http://tinyurl.com/nblw5tj Retrieved 15 January 2014

4. BBC News *'R.I.P The Fat Slags'* http://tinyurl.com/ntcupq3 Retrieved 12 January 2014

5. https://en.wikipedia.org/wiki/File:Alphabet44.jpg Retrieved 13 January 2014

6. Ann Summers - http://www.annsummers.com/page/BraFittingAndInfo Retrieved 27 January 2014

7. Figleaves bra calculator - http://tinyurl.com/pfhp9yg Retrieved 13 January 2014

8. Bravissimo bra fitting video guide http://tinyurl.com/q7dh37b Retrieved 27 January 2014

9. White, Jenny and Scurr, Joanna (2012) *'Evaluation of professional bra fitting criteria for bra selection and fitting in the UK.'* Ergonomics, 55 (6). pp. 704-711. http://tinyurl.com/o38q2dx

10. Power, Marianne, Daily Mail online *'So that's why your bras never fit!'* http://tinyurl.com/798vyyp Retrieved 5 January 2014

REFERENCES

11. http://www.theguardian.com/world/2000/oct/31/gender.uk

12. Seigel, Jessica 'Bent Out Of Shape - *'Why is it so hard to find the perfect bra?'*. http://www.jessicaseigel.com/articles/bra.shtml Retrieved 13 January 2014

13. Daily Telegraph 02 November 2000 http://tinyurl.com/ovza9ez Retrieved 10 January 2014

14. Morris, Desmond. *'The Naked Ape: A Zoologist's Study of the Human Animal'* (Hardback: ISBN 0-07-043174-4; Reprint: ISBN 0-385-33430-3) (1967)

15. Florence Williams' 'Breasts: Natural and Unnatural History' which is available from Amazon http://tinyurl.com/n6gv24a

16. Wikipedia Media Commons Image by Bartholomeus van der Helst (1613–1670) http://tinyurl.com/naz4w6v

17. Wikipedia Media Commons Image http://en.wikipedia.org/wiki/File:FlapperOnShip1929_crop.jpg Retrieved 3 March 2014

18. http://en.wikipedia.org/wiki/Human_penis_size

19. https://en.wikipedia.org/wiki/Ptosis_(breasts) Retrieved 13 January 2014

20. *'Brassiere Support Is A Lie, Say French Scientists'* Popular Science http://tinyurl.com/bsufl7v Retrieved 13 January 2014

21. Singer, Sydney Ross and Grismaijer, Soma *'Dressed To Kill: The Link Between Breast Cancer and Bras'* Avery Publishing Corp. New York 1995 ISBN 0-89529-664-0

22. Ray, Claiborne, 'Bras and Cancer' http://tinyurl.com/o98ujf3 Retrieved 10 January 2014

23. World map showing incidence of breast cancer by country http://tinyurl.com/m977lwq

24. http://en.wikipedia.org/wiki/Body_mass_index Retrieved 27 January 2014

25. Cecchini RS1, Costantino JP, Cauley JA, Cronin WM, Wickerham DL, Land SR, Weissfeld JL, Wolmark N. *'Body mass index and the risk for developing invasive breast cancer among high-risk women in NSABP P-1 and STAR breast cancer prevention trials.'* Cancer Prev Res (Phila). 2012 Apr;5 (4):583-92.

REFERENCES

doi: 10.1158/1940-6207.CAPR-11-0482. Epub 2012 Feb 7. Retrieved 20 February 2014

26. Tracey D. Wade, Gu Zhu, and Nicholas G. Martin *'Body Mass Index and Breast Size in Women: Same or Different Genes?'* http://tinyurl.com/ngctjxp Retrieved 20 February 2014

27. http://www.breastcancercampaign.org/about-breast-cancer/breast-cancer-risk-factors/lifestyle-factors Retrieved 20 February 2014

28. Kusano AS1, Trichopoulos D, Terry KL, Chen WY, Willett WC, Michels KB. Int J Cancer. 2006 Apr 15;118(8):2031-4. 'A prospective study of breast size and premenopausal breast cancer incidence.'

29. Paul Williams, Ph.D., staff scientist, Lawrence Berkeley National Laboratory, Berkeley, Calif.; Leslie Bernstein, Ph.D., professor and director, division of cancer etiology, City of Hope Comprehensive Cancer Center, Duarte, Calif.; Jan. 27, 2014, International Journal of Cancer

30. http://en.wikipedia.org/wiki/Stomach_ulcer#History Retrieved 27 January 2014

31. http://tinyurl.com/q8wb2dx Retrieved 10 March 2014

32. Cancer Research UK http://tinyurl.com/loespwc Retrieved 27 January 2014

33. The James Webb Telescope, Wikipedia. http://tinyurl.com/qd8m2j2 Retrieved 13 January 2014

34. Wikipedia Breast weight http://tinyurl.com/4otkp86 Retrieved 27 January 2014

35. http://en.wikipedia.org/wiki/Blaise_Pascal Retrieved 20 February 2014

36. Moth, David, *'Experiment to measure the force exerted by a bra on the lymphatic system.'* http://www.moth.freeserve.co.uk/page30.html Retrieved 27 January 2014

37. Franzeck UK, Spiegel I, Fischer M, Bortzler C, Stahel HU, Bollinger A. Department of Medicine, University Hospital, Zurich, Switzerland. J Vasc Res 1997 Jul-Aug;34(4):306-11 *'Combined physical therapy for lymphedema evaluated by fluorescence microlymphography and lymph capillary pressure*

REFERENCES

measurements.' Retrieved 13 January 2014

38. Singer, Sydney http://www.killerculture.com/breast-cancer-is-preventable/ Retrieved 13 January 2014

39. CC Hsieh, D Trichopoulos (1991). *'Breast size, handedness and breast cancer risk.'* European Journal of Cancer and Clinical Oncology 27(2):131-135.

40. Komen, Susan G. Blog *'Understanding breast cancer'* http://tinyurl.com/88nwzqp

41. Singer and Grismaijer *'Get It Off!'* (ISCD Press, 2000).

42. Zhang A.Q, Xia J.H, Wang Q, Li W.P, Xu J, Chen Z.Y, Yang J.M (2009). *'Risk factors of breast cancer in women in Guangdong and the countermeasures'*. In Chinese. Nan Fang Yi Ke Da XueXue Bao. 2009 Jul;29(7):1451-3

43. Dr. Marcos Eduardo Quijada Stanovich *'Patologias mamarias generadas por el uso sostenido y seleccion incorrecta del brassier en pacientes que acuden a la consulta de mastologia'* http://tinyurl.com/pjz6f54

44. Cancer Research UK http://tinyurl.com/loespwc

45. Singer and Grismaijer *'Get It Off!'* I.S.C.D. Press (2000) ISBN: 1-930858-01-9

46. http://www.killerculture.com/self-study-center/ Retrieved 27 March 2014

47. http://breathing.com/articles/brassieres-2.htm Retrieved 27 January 2014

48. http://www.theguardian.com/world/2000/oct/31/gender.uk

49. BBC News Online http://news.bbc.co.uk/1/hi/health/998348.stm Retrieved 30 March 2014

50. *'Losing Bra Eases Breast Pain'* Peoples Pharmacy Online http://tinyurl.com/3vl8q86 Retrieved 27 January 2014

51. Wonderbra advert 1994 http://tinyurl.com/ouudjdr Retrieved 13 January 2014

52. http://en.wikipedia.org/wiki/Wonderbra

53. Figleaves bra calculator - http://tinyurl.com/pfhp9yg Retrieved 13 January 2014

REFERENCES

54. Bravissimo bra fitting video guide http://tinyurl.com/q7dh37b Retrieved 27 January 2014

55. Brasize - http://www.brasize.com/ Retrieved 27 January 2014

56. 85b - http://www.85b.org/bra_calc.php Retrieved 27 January 2014

57. Sizeguideuk - http://tinyurl.com/pjnle8u Retrieved 27 January 2014

58. Sizeguide - http://www.sizeguide.net/bra-sizes.html Retrieved 27 January 2014

59. Warner Bra Sizing http://tinyurl.com/ouqkztf

60. La Senza - http://www.lasenza.co.uk/bra-fitting-guide/ Retrieved 29 January 2014

61. Amazon Bra Fitting Guide - http://tinyurl.com/nocd6dp or any other Amazon.co.uk page selling a bra then click on 'Sizing info'. Retrieved 27 January 2014

62. Wikihow (second method) http://www.wikihow.com/Measure-Your-Bra-Size Retrieved 27 January 2014

63. Marks & Spencer bra fitting guide - http://tinyurl.com/o2x2wj5 Retrieved 27 January 2014

64. M&S bra pressure device http://www.openerg.com/brasensor.htm

65. Avon bra fitting guide - http://tinyurl.com/oyopwhp Retrieved 27 January 2014

66. Ample Bosom bra fitting guide - http://www.amplebosom.com/measuring-guide.php Retrieved 27 January 2014

67. Beautiful Lingerie bra fitting guide - http://tinyurl.com/o8kbtf9 Retrieved 27 January 2014

68. Female First bra fitting guide - http://www.femalefirst.co.uk/catalog/sizing-chart.php Retrieved 26 January 2014

69. Bare Necessities - http://tinyurl.com/7zeqrc8 Retrieved 26 January 2014

REFERENCES

70. 85b - http://www.85b.org/bra_calc.php Retrieved 27 January 2014

71. Boobydoo - http://www.boobydoo.co.uk/bra-size-calculator Retrieved 13 January 2014

72. New Look - http://tinyurl.com/m6tazq5 Retrieved 26 January 2014

73. 007b - http://www.007b.com/bra-fitting.php Retrieved 26 January 2014

74. eBay - http://tinyurl.com/mehw7m2 Retrieved 26 January 2014

75. Silk Cocoon - http://tinyurl.com/l7cokhf Retrieved 26 January 2014

76. calculator.net - http://www.calculator.net/bra-size-calculator.html Retrieved 13 January 2014

77. PSLingerie - http://www.pslingerie.co.uk/bra-size-calculator Retrieved 13 January 2014

78. Debenhams - http://tinyurl.com/o84gfb6 Retrieved 13 January 2014

79. mumsnet.com - http://www.mumsnet.com/style-and-beauty/bra-guide Retrieved 13 January 2014

80. wisegeek.org - http://www.wisegeek.org/how-do-i-determine-my-bra-size.htm Retrieved 13 January 2014

81. herroom.com - http://tinyurl.com/nqyuqhp Retrieved 13 January 2014

82. Ann Summers - http://www.annsummers.com/page/BraFittingAndInfo Retrieved 13 January 2014

83. House of Fraser bra fitting guide - http://tinyurl.com/pyywaxf Retrieved 13 January 2014

84. Figleaves bra calculator - http://tinyurl.com/pfhp9yg Retrieved 13 January 2014

85. Fashion World - http://tinyurl.com/nntn99w Retrieved 13 January 2014

86. White, Jenny and Scurr, Joanna (2012) *Evaluation of professional bra fitting criteria for bra selection and fitting in the*

REFERENCES

UK.' Ergonomics, 55 (6). pp. 704-711. http://tinyurl.com/o38q2dx

87. Bravissimo bra fitting video guide http://tinyurl.com/q7dh37b Retrieved 27 January 2014

88. Figleaves bra calculator - http://tinyurl.com/pfhp9yg Retrieved 13 January 2014

89. White, Jenny and Scurr, Joanna (2012) *'Evaluation of professional bra fitting criteria for bra selection and fitting in the UK.'* Ergonomics, 55 (6). pp. 704-711. http://tinyurl.com/o38q2dx

90. Sanders-Steel, Debra *'The Ultimate Bra Fitting Guide'* Outskirts Press Inc. (2013) Available from Amazon

91. White, Jenny and Scurr, Joanna (2012) *'Evaluation of professional bra fitting criteria for bra selection and fitting in the UK.'* Ergonomics, 55 (6). pp. 704-711. http://tinyurl.com/o38q2dx

92. Figleaves bra calculator - http://tinyurl.com/pfhp9yg Retrieved 13 January 2014

93. Bravissimo bra fitting video guide http://tinyurl.com/q7dh37b Retrieved 27 January 2014

94. Power, Marianne, Daily Mail online *'So that's why your bras never fit!'* http://tinyurl.com/798vyyp Retrieved 5 January 2014

95. Wikipedia http://tinyurl.com/ntk3t9r Retrieved 20 February 2014

96. Abraham, Tamara. Daily Mail Online 2 October 2012 http://tinyurl.com/o83j46c

97. 'Gok Wan: Made In China' http://tinyurl.com/p3x2cbd

98. Susan Nethero *'Bra Talk' - Myths and Facts'* Kindle eBook.

99. This Wikipedia and Wikimedia Commons image is from the user Chris 73 and is freely available at http://tinyurl.com/q64bnk2 under the creative commons cc-by-sa 3.0 license.

100. For example see http://tinyurl.com/q92lejy Retrieved 27 January 2014

101. New Scientist 29 March 2014 p 14

102. http://en.wikipedia.org/wiki/File:Lebr03.jpg Retrieved 6 April 2014

REFERENCES

Printed in Great Britain
by Amazon